Change and Development in Specialist Public Health Practice

Change and Development in Specialist Public Health Practice

Siân Griffiths

Immediate Past President
UK Faculty of Public Health
Professor of Public Health
Chinese University of Hong Kong

Allison Thorpe

Project Manager
Thames Valley Strategic Health Authority

and

Jenny Wright

Director
Public Health Resource Unit

Radcliffe Publishing
Oxford • Seattle

Radcliffe Publishing Ltd
18 Marcham Road
Abingdon
Oxon OX14 1AA
United Kingdom

www.radcliffe-oxford.com
Electronic catalogue and worldwide online ordering.

British Library Cataloguing in Publication Data

A catalogue record for this book is available from the British Library.

ISBN 1 85775 697 5

614. GRI

Typeset by Anne Joshua & Associates, Oxford
Printed and bound by TJ International Ltd, Padstow, Cornwall

Contents

Foreword   vi

Preface   vii

About the authors   viii

Glossary of terms   ix

Dedications   xi

Chapter 1
Introduction   1

Chapter 2
What, who and where   13

Chapter 3
Developing a modernised and multidisciplinary public health
specialist workforce   29

Chapter 4
Public health specialist practice in community settings:
primary care and local government   39

Chapter 5
Health protection   57

Chapter 6
Public health in the acute setting   71

Chapter 7
Tools for specialist practice   83

Chapter 8
Looking to the future   103

Index   115

Foreword

This book provides a timely and welcome addition to the public health literature. Its approach demonstrates the ways in which the development of public health practice and delivery have evolved to ensure we have high-quality health improvement and health protection services through a period of dynamic change. It recognises the enormous contribution of our specialist workforce in providing leadership, direction and working with others to improve people's health. I believe that the public health system, in its broadest sense, will find this a useful resource to develop their links into the specialist workforce and their thinking on their own, and colleagues', potential roles in taking forward our challenging public health agenda.

Dr Fiona Adshead
Deputy Chief Medical Officer
Department of Health
May 2005

Preface

This book describes the changing environment of specialist public health practice in England, focusing on the changes since 1997 when the Labour government was elected and the first Minister of Public Health was appointed. Based on a belief that public health is a professional specialism with a unique range of skills that can be applied in different work settings to improve health and protect the public, we have drawn on our recent experiences. These include working with a wide range of public health specialists at national and local level. In particular, we have drawn on the work of the Faculty of Public Health with the Minister of Public Health in early 2004 and a consultation exercise carried out by the Public Health Resource Unit (PHRU) on behalf of the Department of Health as part of the overall consultation exercise for *Choosing Health*. Other work of the Faculty of Public Health has been an important source of information and influence.

With the profile and practice of public health receiving political and popular attention, public health specialists face increasing challenges. These include *Choosing Health* in England with its focus on personalising health, the challenge of reducing health inequalities, the new public health system in Wales and the ban on tobacco smoking in public places in Scotland. Recent years have also seen a resurgence of interest in health protection, not just as a result of the events of September 11 but also in response to newly emergent infections such as severe acute respiratory syndrome (SARS), avian flu and methicillin-resistant *Staphylococcus aureus* (MRSA), and the worrying rate of increase in sexually transmitted diseases. Globally, the costs of major public health threats from HIV/ AIDS, TB and malaria continue to be counted. Against this background, what is expected of public health specialists?

- How well are they able to respond to the challenges on this wide canvas?
- What are the policy drivers and directions of travel?
- What are the priorities if the best is to be made of the opportunities that exist?
- What training is needed?

These are the questions that will be addressed in this book.

Siân Griffiths
Allison Thorpe
Jenny Wright
May 2005

About the authors

Professor Siân Griffiths FPH FRCP OBE is the immediate Past President of the UK Faculty of Public Health. She has held a range of positions at all levels of the NHS in the UK in academic and service departments, most recently as Consultant in Public Health at Thames Valley Strategic Health Authority and Senior Clinical Lecturer in the Department of Public Health at Oxford University. She is currently the Professor of Public Health and Director of the School of Public Health at the Chinese University of Hong Kong.

Allison Thorpe BSc (Hons) MRIPH is employed by the Thames Valley Strategic Health Authority. She has recently completed a secondment to the NHSU, focusing on developing the public health workstreams within the organisation, and will be moving to the Department of Health in the near future. Her career in public health has given her experience in project roles at local and national levels. She is currently in the final stages of a Masters in Public Health at Oxford Brookes University.

Jenny Wright MA (Oxon) MSc MPhil FFPH is an accredited Specialist in Public Health. She has a social work, health services research and planning background before moving to public health. She is currently Director of the Public Health Resource Unit which undertakes public health service, project and development work for Thames Valley PCTs and SHA. For the last few years she has been involved in a number of national projects associated with the development of public health specialists and is also Chair of the Faculty of Public Health's Specialist Development Committee.

Glossary of terms

ADsPH	Association of Directors of Public Health
BAMM	British Association of Medical Managers
CCDC	consultant in communicable disease
CDSC	Communicable Disease Surveillance Centre
CEO	chief executive officer
CHRE	Council for Healthcare Regulatory Excellence
CMO	Chief Medical Officer
CPD	continuing professional development
DPH	director of public health
EEA	European Economic Area
EU	European Union
FEW	Food Environment Water Laboratory
FPH	Faculty of Public Health
GDC	General Dental Council
GDP	gross domestic product
GMC	General Medical Council
GMS	general medical services
GP	general practitioner
HCC	Healthcare Commission
HEA	health equity audit
HIA	health impact assessment
HOADS	heads of academic departments of medical schools
HP	health protection
HPA	Health Protection Agency
IOM	Institute of Medicine
KSF	Knowledge and Skills Framework
LAA	local area agreement
LARS	local and regional services
LDP	local delivery plan
LPSA	local public service agreements
LSP	local strategic partnership
MOsH	medical officers of health
MPH	minister of public health
MRSA	methicillin-resistant *Staphylococcus aureus*
NHS	National Health Service
NHSU	National Health Service University
NIHCE	National Institute for Health and Clinical Excellence
NILSI	National Institute for Learning Skills and Innovation
NMC	Nursing and Midwifery Council
NPfIT	National Programme for Information Technology

NSF	National Service Framework
OPM	Office for Public Management
PCG	primary care group
PCT	primary care trust
PHO	public health observatory
PHRU	public health resource unit
PMETB	Postgraduate Medical and Education Training Board
PMS	personal medical services
PSA	public service agreement
QOF	Quality and Outcomes Framework
R&D	research and development
RAE	research assessment exercise
RCGP	Royal College of General Practitioners
SARS	severe acute respiratory syndrome
SHA	strategic health authority
STA	Specialist Training Authority
STI	sexually transmitted infections

Dedications

This book is dedicated to the members of the Faculty of Public Health whose experiences and wisdom we hope we have reflected in these pages.

And for my long suffering proof readers: my husband Graham, and my children Andrew, Christopher and Teryn. I promise I will think about it a lot more before I agree to do anything like this again!   **AT**

And to the staff in the Public Health Resource Unit for their time and support.

Introduction

Introduction

> **Learning point**
>
> - An introduction to the historical, political and health policy context within which specialist public health professionals operate.

The specialist public health profession in England has undergone continuous and significant changes since the publication of *Saving Lives: our healthier nation* by the incoming Labour government's first Minister of Public Health in 1997.[1] Followed by the Acheson report on inequalities, the NHS Plan and the reports of Derek Wanless[2,3] and amidst the changing organisational structures of the healthcare system, specialists have regrouped and faced the challenges posed. In this book we take stock of the context, practice and future challenges to be faced.

Who are specialists in public health?

For the purpose of this book we have taken a definition for public health specialists based on current practice: those who reach the specified competencies as recognised by the Faculty of Public Health and associated registering bodies. This definition is inclusive of all groups reaching the required standards to practice as a specialist, independent of previous professional backgrounds.

The history of public health specialists

It is often helpful to have a thread to follow, and this thread is provided by the story of the Medical Officer of Health. The history of public health in England dates back to the work of Edwin Chadwick, who in his well-known *Report on the Sanitary Condition of the Labouring Population* made the recommendation:

> *that for the general means necessary to prevent disease, it would be good economy to appoint a district medical officer . . . with the securities of special qualifications and responsibilities to initiate sanitary measures.*[4]

This recommendation led to the appointment in 1847 in Liverpool of the first Medical Officer of Health, William Duncan. Duncan was inspired and inspiring. When cholera struck in 1832 he had observed, as a physician, greater numbers of deaths among the poor and overcrowded than among the better off and well housed, an observation recorded in an article he wrote for his local newspaper. A few years later in 1840 his evidence to the House of Commons Select Committee on the Health of Towns described the appalling conditions of many of the workers who had flocked to the city in the industrial revolution. He described the conditions of the one in eight of the population who lived in cellars, many with up to 30 in the same room. No wonder the life expectancy was 19 years compared to the 36.5 years a man could expect to live in Wiltshire.

The improvements pioneered by Duncan, including better sanitary conditions and housing, better drainage, clean water and waste disposal, led to an improvement of six-and-a-half years in life expectancy over a period of 15 years.[5]

To quote Chave:

> Duncan was a trail blazer who, working very largely single handed and with very limited resources, pointed the way along the path of sanitary reform and health improvement which his successors were to follow through the remainder of the century and even after.
>
> He was at once public watchdog and accuser, he was adviser and initiator, he was educator and protector (p. 35).[6]

This was very much the spirit urged on modern day Directors of Public Health by Lord Hunt in his speech in 2001 when he explained the implications of the latest government changes within *Shifting the Balance of Power*:[7,8]

> So, let me make it clear that, in future, the engine of public health delivery will be at the front line around the primary care trust. Every primary care trust will have a director of public health and support team. These directors of public health will be board level appointments working at the heart of the new organisations. The focus of their activity will be on local neighbourhoods and communities leading and driving programmes to improve health and reduce inequalities. They will also play a powerful role in forging partnerships with, and influencing, all local agencies to ensure the widest possible participation in the health and health care agenda.
>
> The director of public health will not be a remote, strategic figure – she or he will be well known, respected and credible with local people – particularly those in the most deprived communities, local authorities, general practitioners and other local clinicians.
>
> This generation of directors of public health will be from a variety of backgrounds not only medical. This reform offers an opportunity to make multi-disciplinary public health a reality. The process of training,

accreditation and appointment will need to be rigorously quality-assured as the responsibilities of this position are substantial.

Although the nineteenth century legislation to create medical officers of health (MOsH) was passed, it took many years for appointments to be made. Things became more complicated with the 1872 and 1875 Public Health Acts when urban and rural authorities were created and all had to have MOsH – in all a total of 1000 were needed. Capacity, as ever, was stretched by organisational reform. The solution was piecemeal. Many appointments were part-time and often token. The majority of appointees were clinicians with an interest, and very few full-time appointments were made.

Chave posed three important questions for MOsH at the time, which may well resonate with us now:

- **status**: should they be specialists with qualifications?
- **salary**: should they be full-time with local government, and therefore salaried and not reliant on income from other aspects of medical practice?
- **security**: should they have security of tenure, thus allowing them to advocate for their population and not be dismissible on the whim of any of the locally elected councillors?[6]

It took 60 years for these issues to be resolved. As the role developed in the latter part of the 19th century it became increasing clear there was a specialty concerned with sanitary science. Courses were set up in universities – first in Dublin, then Cambridge. The branch of the medical profession was formally recognised in 1886 by the General Medical Council (GMC) who registered those with diplomas in public health, sanitary medicine or state medicine. The need for a specialist qualification was recognised when in 1888 the Local Government Act specified that MOsH of any district of population greater than 50 000 needed to hold the diploma in public health.

The role that these early MOsH were expected to play was in line with implementing the 1875 sanitary code. They were expected to take responsibility for ten key areas which included clean water, preventing pollution, suppressing communicable disease, and food inspection.

With the dawn of the 20th century there came an understanding of the nature of bacteriology and with it the opportunity not only for immunisation but also for the development of drug therapies based on scientific understanding. Emphasis shifted away from the environmental focus of the sanitary code to a personalised health service providing, for example, school medicals and health visiting.

The first half of the 20th century saw the development of personal preventive services with maternal and child welfare a public health priority. The 1902 Midwives Act, the 1906 provision of school meals legislation, the founding of the school medical service in 1907 and the Maternity and Child Welfare Acts of 1918 demonstrate this shift to an investment in midwifery, health visiting and school nursing as part of the community-based public health service. The growth of personal health services was followed by the introduction of mass vaccination and immunisation and an increased emphasis on disease prevention. During the same period the 1929 Local Government Act increased hospital resources of county and borough councils, and in 1948 the National Health Service (NHS) was introduced to establish 'a comprehensive health service to secure the improvement in the physical and mental health of the people . . . and the prevention, diagnosis and treatment of illness'.

The health services were then run as a tripartite service – local government public health services, general practice and administered hospitals. Initially MOsH stayed with local government. To quote Rivett:

> By 1968 MOsH had a smoothly running empire, managing community nursing service, social work services, the aftercare of people who were mentally ill or handicapped, the ambulances and the child and school health services.[9]

These services continued to be provided by local government until 1974 when community health services were created within the NHS. Locally each district then had an NHS-employed district community physician who, while inheriting part of the MOH role as well as medical administration, lost the leadership of social services and the organisational position within local government. The professions of social work and environmental health took on their own momentum.

This arrangement fractured the relationship of specialists with those influencing the broader determinants of health, and subsequent reorganisations saw the increasing identification of public health specialists with NHS managerial structures.[10,11] Other parts of the profession continued to develop their separate identities within individual structures.

Outside the planning/management role, the locus of public health practice lay within health promotion, infectious disease control, civil service or academia. Relationships with community-based public health practitioners such as health visitors, school nurses, community development workers and environmental health officers were weakened. Public health specialists became associated with the commissioning function in the early 1990s as the internal market of purchasers and providers linked the newly designated directors of public health and their teams firmly to the purchaser's side of the split. While this had the advantage of public health being located on the management team within district health authorities, the organisation which had the resources as well as population health responsibilities, this was outweighed by the disadvantage of isolation from clinicians, communities and local authorities. There was no unification into a common purpose.

Many in the public health community were left wishing to promote a more coherent focus for public health which addressed root causes of ill-health and was not tied so closely to the vagaries of management structures for delivering health services.

Just as the early MOsH had been advocates not just observers, engaged in local decision making, publishing annual independent public health reports, so too modern specialists wanted to redress the balance of the move toward health service management. In addition, the trend within academic public health to focus on epidemiology rather than closer working with service public health was also an area of tension. As Francis had noted:

> *epidemiology is not enough . . . we must recover the ph attitude of seeing clinical medicine and microbiology as important scientific bases of its practice of prevention (p. 155).*[11]

Where does this leave us?

Following the election of the Labour government in 1997 there was a shift not only within the context but also within the practice of specialists in public health.

A renewed emphasis on the social determinants of health, poor housing, lack of educational opportunity, bad working conditions and poverty created a climate in which it was now permissible to talk of health inequalities rather than coyly referring to 'variations'.[12] It was no longer a climate in which the events surrounding the Black Report would be repeated – publication of a report on health inequalities in what can be best described as a 'limited edition' with 260 duplicated copies of the report made available in the week of the August bank holiday, and then shelved overnight.

The new context of practice was set by the white paper on public health, *Saving Lives: our healthier nation* which built on the previous *Health of the Nation*.[1,13] In the introduction the prime minister highlighted three complementary levels of action to improve health:

- individuals and their families taking action for themselves
- communities working together in partnership
- government acting to address the major determinants through policy on areas such as jobs, housing, education.

The key elements of *Saving Lives* included:

- a focus on reducing inequalities with an increased awareness of the wider determinants of health and the health responsibilities of bodies and organisations other than the NHS

- targets and pathways for reducing the burden of disease from major killers of coronary heart disease, accidents and cancer as well as the need to reduce mental ill-health
- tools such as health impact assessment and collection of data by public health observatories to monitor health
- setting standards and developing the specialist and practitioner work-force.[1]

The theme of addressing health inequalities, as highlighted by Black, has continued to be reflected in health policy.[12] In 1998 Sir Donald Acheson's independent inquiry into inequalities in health was published, making 39 recommendations of which only three related to the NHS.[14] The inquiry identified three key actions to reduce inequalities:

- policy evaluation for the impact on health of inequalities
- high priority given to health of families and young children
- reduction of income inequalities and improvement of living standards of poor households.

Some of the immediate responses from government included:

- the investment in SureStart
- the Healthy Schools Programme
- a focus on reduction of teenage pregnancy: the targets for the teenage pregnancy strategy also direct work to many of the most deprived communities. Much of the work is this area already rests on the recognition that the risk of becoming a teenage mother for girls from the poorest families is almost ten times higher than for those from the richest families
- the publication of the *Smoking Kills* white paper, with its focus on reducing smoking in under 16s: smoking cessation services have been targeted on the lowest income sectors with free nicotine replacement therapy
- across-government policy initiatives through the Social Exclusion Unit/ Neighbourhood Renewal: initiatives have addressed many of the issues raised in the inquiry[15]
- rapid access chest pain clinics provide access to diagnosis for heart disease, starting in areas of highest need and lowest income
- the cervical smear programme has developed local initiatives to promote screening in minority ethnic communities
- new investment in primary care is targeted in low-income areas
- the five-a-day programme has been established to develop skills so that people are better able to produce, prepare and cook fruit and vegetables, and it also promotes access to fruit and vegetables in deprived areas, targeting communities poorly served at present

- many children are now receiving a free piece of fruit each school day through the national school fruit scheme
- lottery funding through the New Opportunities Fund has created Healthy Living Centres in the most deprived parts of the UK.

While these initiatives reflect a policy shift towards public health, this shift is often seen as too little and with too low a profile. The strategic direction for the NHS set out in *The NHS Plan* included a chapter on addressing health inequalities, but this was separated from the major thrust to improve health services which was to receive the lion's share of new resources.[16] Policy documents followed such as *Tackling Health Inequalities: summary of the 2002 cross cutting review* and *Tackling Health Inequalities: a programme for action* with cross-government responsibilities mapped out.[17,18]

More recently the second iteration of the *NHS Plan, The NHS improvement Plan: putting people at the heart of public services*, once again recognises that health as well as health services is the business of the NHS: 'the promotion of health and prevention of ill health will assume a much more important role in the work of the NHS' (p. 42).[19]

Some of this has been picked up with the current performance management workstreams for primary care – for example the Balanced Score card system of assessing primary care trust (PCT) performance details some key targets around substance misuse and smoking cessation. The future performance management system for PCTs and hospital trusts, recently outlined by the Healthcare Commission has also a specific domain for public health.[20] The future planning targets also have a specific domain for public health – all of which indicates that the climate is changing.[21,22]

While this list of policy intentions may seem impressive, it has been generally accepted that not enough has been done to deflect the criticism that the focus of the NHS and its resources is disproportionately downstream on patients, not upstream on prevention.

The most vocal, and most influential, proponent of this criticism is Derek Wanless. Commissioned by the Treasury in 2002 to review the future spending needs of the NHS, his first report *Securing Our Future: taking a long term view* highlighted the need to invest in reducing demand by enhancing the promotion of health and disease prevention.[2] His second report takes forward this theme and analyses how to achieve the 'fully engaged' scenario, proposed as the best use of resources for improving future health of the population. Frustration with continual analysis and lack of follow-up action is reflected throughout the report which quotes Hunter:

> *Health policy has remained biased towards the 'National Sickness Service' and towards the medical model of avoiding ill health and disease . . . so in spite of numerous policy initiatives being directed*

towards public health, they have not resulted in a rebalancing of policy away from health care. The report recommends that after many years of reviews and government policy documents, with little change on the ground, the key challenge now is delivery and implementation not further discussion.[23]

The response from the Department of Health to the Wanless criticisms was to announce, just in advance of the publication of *Securing Health*, a consultation on a future white paper – *Choosing Health*.[24] Based around questions about lifestyle – diet, physical activity, sexual health, tobacco, alcohol – the consultation focused on engaging a wide range of stakeholders in the debate about how to improve health. One of the key issues was the balance between what individuals can do themselves and what actions, for example banning smoking in public places, need to be taken by government. Focus was also given to the importance of building social capital in communities, particularly through investment in those who are more deprived.

The latest white paper, *Choosing Health*, takes forward the health improvement agenda, focusing on promoting opportunities for individuals to take responsibility for their own health and establishing a series of programmes of work in key areas such as tackling obesity through better nutrition and more physical activity, reducing tobacco smoking, promoting mental health, action on alcohol abuse and improving sexual health services and education. Commitment to building up the infrastructure needed to underpin these programmes includes a programme of work to strengthen the public health workforce. The overall strategy will be to build capacity at all levels, including increasing capacity and developing skills in public health specialists. Recognition of the diversity of the multidisciplinary workforce, the need for generic and specialist standards of practice and for new ways of working are signposted. In particular, public health specialists will be expected to be competent to lead and deliver key health improvement services, to be competent to work with communities and to tackle inequalities. The skills needed will include the ability to communicate effectively and to understand what motivates individuals to change their behaviour. Commitment to increasing capacity reflects the need to increase public health input to undergraduate curriculae for healthcare workers, for postgraduate pathways to specialist practice, for flexible career options and for engaging managers. Further emphasis is given to developing and sustaining academic careers as well as creating national and international links, including those with the HPA and other agencies with public health roles.

Public health has now become everybody's business. But with this increasing profile there is also the risk it will be nobody's business to ensure a co-ordinated, comprehensive response. This must be the role of specialists – but how will they respond to the challenges of:

- growing interest
- wider engagement
- new expectations of personalising health improvement
- a higher profile
- and the need to address inequalities and deliver better health for all?

References

1 Department of Health (1999) *Saving Lives: our healthier nation*. Department of Health, London.
2 HM Treasury (2002) *Securing Our Future: taking a long term view*. HM Treasury, London.
3 HM Treasury (2004) *Securing Good Health for the Whole Population*. HM Treasury, London.
4 Chadwick E (1842) *Report on the Sanitary Condition of the Labouring Population*. Edinburgh University Press, Edinburgh. This edition published in 1965.
5 Ashton J (1997) *Health in Our Time: The William Henry Duncan Memorial Lectures*. Carnegie Publishing, Preston.
6 Warren M and Francis H (1987) *Recalling the Medical Officer of Health: writings by Sidney Chave*. King Edward's Hospital Fund for London, King's Fund, London.
7 Hunt P (2001) *First Annual Faculty of Public Health Lecture*. Royal College of Physicians, London.
8 Department of Health (2001) *Shifting the Balance of Power in England*. Department of Health, London.
9 Rivett GC (1998) *From Cradle to Grave: fifty years of the NHS*. King's Fund, London.
10 Holland WW and Stewart S (1998) *Public Health: the vision and the challenge*. Nuffield Trust (Rock Carling Fellowship 1997), London, cited in Hunter DJ (2003) *Public Health Policy*. Polity Press, Cambridge.
11 Francis H (1987) Towards community medicine: the British experience. In: Bennett AE (ed.) *Recent Advances in Community Medicine 1*. Churchill Livingstone, Edinburgh.
12 Department of Health (1980) *Report of the Working Group on Inequalities in Health – the 'Black Report'*. Department of Health, London.
13 Department of Health (1992) *Health of the Nation*. Department of Health, London.
14 Department of Health (1988) *Public Health in England. Report of the Committee of Inquiry into the Future Development of the Public Health Function*. Department of Health, London.
15 Social Exclusion Unit (2001) *A New Commitment to Neighbourhood Renewal: National Strategy and Action Plan*. HMSO, London.
16 Department of Health (2000) *The NHS Plan*. Department of Health, London.
17 Department of Health (2002) *Tackling Health Inequalities: summary of the 2002 cross cutting review*. Department of Health, London.
18 Department of Health (2003) *Tackling Health Inequalities: a programme for action*. Department of Health, London.

19 Department of Health (2004) *The NHS Improvement Plan: putting people at the heart of public services*. Department of Health, London.

20 Healthcare Commission (2004) *Assessment for Improvement: our approach*. Healthcare Commission, London.

21 Department of Health (2004) *National Standards, Local Action: health and social care standards and planning framework (2005/06–2007/08)*. Department of Health, London.

22 Department of Health (2004) *Standards for Better Health: health care standards for services under the NHS*. Department of Health, London.

23 Hunter DJ (2003) *Public Health Policy*. Polity Press, Cambridge.

24 Department of Health (2004) *Choosing Health Consultation Document*. Department of Health, London.

25 Department of Health (2004) *Choosing Health: making healthy choices easier*. Department of Health, London.

What, who and where

What, who and where

Learning points

- How do we define the specialist role?
- What are specialists' core skills and experience?
- Where do they practise? The different levels within NHS, government and government office, health protection, university and academic settings.

What: a definition of public health

The historical origins of the public health movement led to a set of characteristics which are reflected in the *Alma Ata Declaration* of Health for All and in the *Ottawa Charter*.[1,2] These seminal papers emphasise wellbeing – not just absence of disease – as the basis of public health, stressing that it is not only the impact of individual behaviours that influences the health of the population, but also more importantly the effects of social, economic, political and environmental factors. To be effective, public health needs, therefore, to:

- be population based
- emphasise collective responsibility for health, its protection and disease prevention
- recognise the key role of the state, linked to a concern for the underlying socio-economic and wider determinants of health, as well as disease
- have a multidisciplinary basis, which incorporates quantitative, as well as qualitative methods
- emphasise partnerships with all of those who contribute to the health of the population – including individuals, communities, voluntary groups and the business sector.

There is no internationally agreed definition of public health, rather variations on this Ottawa theme. In the United States, the Institute of Medicine defines public health as:

> *what we as a society do collectively to assure the conditions in which people can be healthy.*[3]

In Canada, the newly created Public Health Agency, describes public health in the following way:

> *Unlike health care, which focuses on the individual, public health targets the entire population by identifying threats to the health of Canadians and developing programs and initiatives to address these threats and keep Canadians healthy.*[4]

In the UK, following the Acheson review into public health in 1988,[5] the most frequently employed definition, building on that of Winslow,[6] has been that public health is:

> *the science and art of preventing disease, prolonging life and promoting, protecting and improving health through the organised efforts of society.*

Wanless in his second report that looks at public health suggested an adaptation:

> *the science and art of preventing disease, prolonging life and promoting health through the organised efforts and informed choices of society, organisations, public and private, communities and individuals.*[7]

This refinement was suggested to reflect the policy shift towards personalising the public health agenda. In line with the increasing emphasis placed on individual choice within health policy, it tends to polarise the debate between individual choice and state intervention, highlighting the tension about how much can be achieved by governments without being accused of 'nanny statism', and how much needs to be left to individual choice. Our opinion is that public health needs to recognise the interaction between government and the individual, but also reflect the important role of the community and of social endeavour in promoting health. This balance is perhaps best represented by the well-known diagram which scopes the horizons of specialist practice, demonstrating the need not only for technical skills to support individuals in promoting healthy choices but also for skills to influence the broader determinants which impact on the health of populations (*see* Figure 2.1).

One model of practice that has been proposed through specialist organisations such as the Association of Directors of Public Health (ADsPH) is based on three domains of practice. The three domains are interrelated but distinct aspects of public health practice and provide a framework to describe both the services to be delivered and also the roles and responsibilities of those delivering them, particularly the core skills, knowledge and competencies that are needed (*see* Figure 2.2).

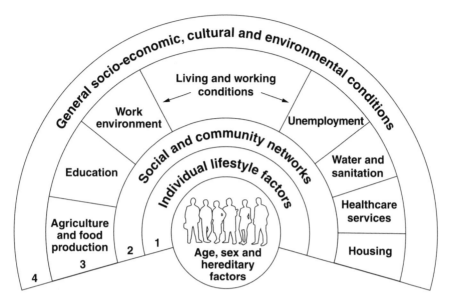

Figure 2.1: The main determinants of health. (Source: Whitehead and Dahlgren, 1991.[8])

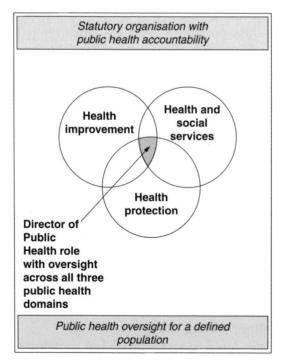

Figure 2.2: The three domains of public health. (Source: Association of Directors of Public Health, 2004.[9])

The three domains reflect the historical roots of public health. They are:

- health improvement which draws heavily on the local government roots of the profession
- health protection which incorporates the response not only to infectious disease but to environmental and bioterrorist threats
- health service quality improvement which develops the territory claimed by doyens such as Archie Cochrane, the exponent of clinical effectiveness, as well as incorporating the historic responsibility for re-engagement in planning and managing services.

In a recent survey of primary care trust (PCT) directors of public health (DPHs) in the spring of 2004 as part of the consultation on *Choosing Health,* most DPHs (88% of those in our survey) agreed that their role was to take an overview across the three domains.[10] Other specialists may have special expertise in one or other domain. For example, consultants in communicable disease control (CCDCs) will work mainly within the domain of health protection, while health promotion specialists work within health improvement. All specialists will however be expected to share basic competence in core areas.

The three domains provide a map for identifying the relative contributions of the different groups involved in the public health workforce. Each domain needs to be supported by public health intelligence and information, which some see as a potential fourth domain of practice, by academic research and by a clear strategy for developing the workforce.[11]

Delivering public health

While the three domains help to organise public health tasks across different sectors, there is value in considering activity as part of a system of service delivery. Characteristics of such a system would include those detailed in Box 2.1.

Box 2.1: Characteristics of public health service delivery[11]

- Working within national policy frameworks
- Working at all population levels including with national public health agencies
- Delivering comprehensive public health programmes for populations, including vulnerable groups, to improve and protect health
- Being an integral part of primary care
- Having a DPH in each locality/geographic area

- Having locally organised multidisciplinary public health teams made up of specialists, practitioners, and those with an interest including voluntary and community groups and community advocates, who are all part of *managed* public health networks
- Being supported by timely, accurate and accessible public health information
- Being performance-managed for process, output and outcome including reaching targets
- Having local discretion about priorities and methods of delivery
- Being based on strong partnerships with communities and local government and the voluntary sector
- Framing and monitoring activities through DPH annual reports which provide an independent assessment of the health of the local population, supporting health equity audits and health impact assessments
- Ensuring action on key public health issues is reflected in the plans of partners as well as the NHS local delivery plans
- Being underpinned by support from academic colleagues

Who are the specialist public health workforce and where do they work?

In his review of the public health function published in 2000, the Chief Medical Officer (CMO) of England described three levels for the workforce (*see* Figure 2.3):[12]

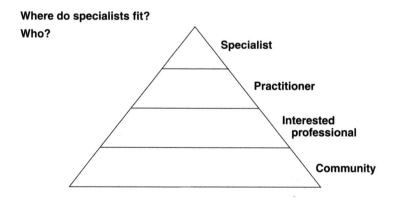

Recommended ratio: 25 specialists per million population by 2006

Figure 2.3: The public health workforce.[13]

- **public health specialists**: consultants and specialists in public health who work at a strategic or senior management level or at a senior level of scientific expertise to influence the health of the whole population or of a selected community. These professionals have specialist knowledge and skills, have met the required Faculty of Public Health standards for higher specialist training, or equivalent, and their core task is public health. They can work at different levels and in different environments (*see* Table 2.1). The ability to manage change, to lead public health programmes and to work across organisational boundaries is crucial for this group
- **public health practitioners**: those who spend a major part, or in some cases all of their time in public health or preventative practice during their hands-on work with individuals or groups of people. This group includes health visitors, environmental health officers, community development workers and those who use research, information, public health science or health promotion skills in specific public health fields. They may be involved in a wide variety of activities, including school health checks, advice on falls prevention, operational delivery of public health programmes, etc
- **the wider workforce**: who have a role in health improvement and reducing inequalities, e.g. chief executives, teachers, local business leaders, social workers, transport engineers, housing officers, other local government staff and members of the voluntary sector, health service managers.

The recent government public health white paper *Choosing Health* expands the third category to include health advocates and advisers, drawn from communities themselves.[14] These advisers, designated as trainers, will be given skills to assist them in providing advice to anyone who feels they need support to develop a healthier lifestyle. The NHS workforce also represents an important group amongst those interested in improving health. Staff in the NHS need to be supported to both understand and value their own health, and to be able to communicate key messages to patients and others they come into contact with through their work. These messages need to be based on evidence and communicated in ways that are most effective to support people who wish to adopt healthier behaviours. To meet this challenge, health improvement will be highlighted in induction programmes.

All those with an interest in developing public health skills will be provided with the necessary opportunities to develop these skills and be supported in effecting change. The Wanless report stresses the need for a strategic approach, including towards the development of specialists in public health, who are a very small but essential part of the overall workforce.[7]

The specialist public health workforce

Specialists have diverse roles within the public health system. This is illustrated in the framework in Figure 2.4 and described in Table 2.1.

Where?

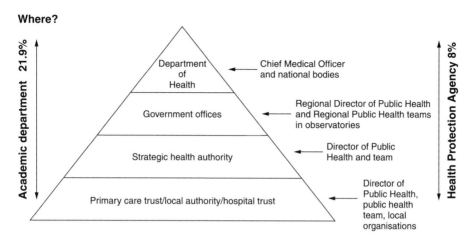

Figure 2.4: Distribution of the specialist workforce.[13]

Particular difficulties have been faced by the specialist public health workforce in England because they have been so closely tied into the organisational structures of the NHS. The consequence of sequential reorganisations over recent years has been employment instability and role changes (*see* Chapter 1). This has inevitably weakened and fragmented the specialist profession and its relationships with others in public health, not only in the NHS but in other sectors. With the renewed focus on public health, the professional aspects of the role of public health specialist are being more clearly delineated. A major step has been to develop multidisciplinary specialists who share equivalent status to the doctors who previously dominated specialist practice.

Currently the distribution of specialist skills across the country is patchy, and in most places falls well below the recommendations of the Faculty of Public Health Workforce Survey of 2003 which identified large geographical variations in the specialist workforce and a shortfall in specialist practice.

> *If each region were to achieve the same as the highest this would require an increase of approximately 20% of trainees, 25% more consultants and specialists, and 50% more public health academics in the UK. If the rates in London were to be applied, these numbers would be even higher (p. 4).*[13]

It recommended that specialist capacity be increased to a norm of 25 per million by 2006.

Over time, as the multidisciplinary nature of specialist public health practice develops, a clearer identity for different specialist groups – for example environmental scientists, nutritional experts, psychologists – will expand the range of posts and environments where specialists can work and the workforce is needed.

Table 2.1: Specialist roles at the different levels of the public health system.

Level of practice/employing agency	Functions	Specialists engaged in delivery	Further discussion
Department of Health	• Develop and implement national health policy • Link with other government departments • National overview through Chief Medical Officer's newsletters and annual report • Centrally fund relevant programmes • Oversee performance delivery	• Chief Medical Officer • Deputy Chief Medical Officer • Public health team • Special health authorities • National Institute for Health and Clinical Excellence (NIHCE)	Cross-cutting theme
Regional government offices	• Lead teams that influence wider determinants including transport, housing, employment and education through working with regional and local government • Lead development/implementation of regional frameworks for health • Ensure effective contribution to local strategic partnerships • Responsible for ensuring performance improvement information from all sectors relevant to reducing health inequalities is acted on by strategic health authorities • Commission regional public health training schemes • Commission the public health observatory • Strategic approach to research and development capacity and activity	• Regional director of public health • Regional public health team • Public health observatories and their teams • Cancer Registry staff	Chapter 2
Strategic health authorities	• Performance management of PCTs and trusts through monitoring, improvement and management mechanisms • Implementation of national screening programmes • Public health capacity development • Research governance systems • Integrate national priorities into local planning mechanisms	• Director of Public Health • Specialists, medical and other • Public health team	Chapter 2

Hospital trusts	• Epidemiological skills • Management skills • Information skills • Develop acute trust contribution to workforce health, corporate citizen role of trust	• Consultants/specialists in public health • Epidemiologists • Microbiologists	Chapter 6
PCTs and local authorities	• Lead the health improvement agenda, working in partnership e.g. local strategic partnerships • Commission and provide primary care and other health services • Local level health protection • Robust clinical governance systems • Implement, commission and manage programmes • Contribute to networks to support PCT activity • Manage, support and develop staff • Promote wider understanding of health needs • Partnership work with other agencies to deliver health agenda • Annual report • Commission health promotion information	• DPHs • Consultants • Public health specialists • Joint posts with local authorities • Public health dental/pharmacist specialists • Health improvement specialists • Health informatics/intelligence specialists	Chapter 4
Academic community	• Teaching: there are many Masters in Public Health courses but no national accreditation • Research: primary and secondary analysis, dissemination of evidence • Support capacity building • Contribute actively to local partnerships	• Universities • Academic public health departments • Research staff • Multidisciplinary workforce Traditionally part of the medical disciplines, the broader definition of public health has opened up opportunities for other disciplines – although service may be slower to implement • Masters in Public Health students	Chapter 2
Health Protection Agency	• Health protection expertise, advise, resource and management • Research engagement	• Local and regional services • Communicable Disease Surveillance Centre – national role • Chemical division • National Radiation Protection Board • Emergency response division	Chapter 5

Academic public health

Defining academic public health is complex because of the diversity of interests from within biomedical and social sciences, amongst others which could be included. The recent report by the Wellcome Foundation recognised this:

> The term 'public health sciences' is a broad church. It is characterised by diversity, with a variety of disciplines involved in public health research, and both quantitative and qualitative approaches to the evaluation of public health interventions.[15]

Given this breadth it is disappointing that one of the areas acknowledged as suffering professional neglect has been academic public health, as described in the survey by the Council of Heads of Medical Schools which made it clear that academic public health (medicine) faces severe problems.[16] The report shows that between 2000 and 2003, public health has been the worst affected of all medical specialties, losing 32% of all posts. When this is put alongside the drop in pathology, a loss of 25%, this is particularly harmful for the future of academic health protection. Changes by grade in the same time period showed a loss of 20% of professorial posts, 22% of readers/senior lecturers and 59% of lecturers. In addition public health medicine has lost the highest percentage of funding from outside sources.

The Wellcome report published in 2004 reflected the concern about the weakness of academic public health, highlighting that links between academic and service public health are weak.[15] Academic public health careers have suffered in recent years, badly affected not only by values within the research assessment exercise (RAE) which fail to reward service-related work, but also by all the structural changes following the establishment of PCTs (in 2002). Financial support for public health sciences comes from a variety of governmental, research council and charitable resources, and there is currently no overarching strategic framework to decide upon priorities or relative roles. Given this analysis the main recommendations of the Wellcome report were that academic public health sciences would be strengthened by:

- establishing a national strategy for public health sciences to underpin the future strategic direction of public health sciences as a multi-disciplinary endeavour
- implementing a structured programme of long-term investment in training at all levels
- addressing the structural barriers to partnership working between the academic sector and NHS colleagues

- reviewing and streamlining the regulatory framework for research to support population-based research
- addressing the perceived problems between data protection and use of population-based data.[15]

When the Wellcome report recommendations were tested against the views of the heads of academic departments of medical schools (HOADS) in the *Choosing Health* consultation (spring 2004), they were all strongly supported.[10]

At a time when the UK health service is being refocused towards the promotion of good health and the prevention of illness there was support for an overarching national strategy to secure the future of the public health sciences. The strategy should:[10]

- 'be informed by evidence on the size and nature of health problems and the availability of cost-effective interventions'
- 'put an end to the current problem of one policy undermining another'
- 'ensure that research is relevant to an agreed national strategy and health policy'
- 'be under the leadership of a centralised strategy committee with commissioning and responsive modes'
- be multidisciplinary in nature
- involve service users, service providers, researchers and the community
- be relevant to both policymakers and practitioners.

Commentators agreed that research groups should be multidisciplinary and involve disciplines such as epidemiology, biostatistics, health economics, health psychology, anthropology and sociology in order to evaluate public health interventions. Other potential disciplines that could be included were geographers, social and public policy researchers and public health historians.

Since the public health sciences are seriously under-resourced, the national framework needs to be matched by a structured programme of long-term investment in workforce development at all levels – undergraduate, postgraduate, research fellow, lecturer, senior lecturer and professor – to strengthen the infrastructure. This would involve commitment from the higher education funding councils, the Department of Health, the NHS and research funding bodies to supporting academic posts. In particular younger members of staff need succession planning. Such a programme would also have a major and equally important impact on the 'non-academic' institutions that are required to improve public health and commission research.

Partnership between the universities and NHS public health needs to be re-established through joint training programmes, joint posts, formal agreements such as the commissioning of research, evaluations and reviews of public health prevention programmes.

Comments included:

> *This joint work should be given priority and not seen as an added extra that university and service public health staff are expected to do on top of other demands on their time.*

Barriers to re-establishing links included the RAE criteria, differences in service and academic cultures, the structure of the NHS, and the need to take a developmental approach for training programmes:

> *Commissioning of research by the local NHS is problematic for universities as it can rarely cover the full costs of the research and rarely ends in publications which can contribute to the RAE, so they are a considerable net drain on resources.*

> *The partnership is critical but there also needs to an appreciation of the two very different cultures, environments and time scales. Universities focus on long-term, generalisable research and evaluations, while the NHS focuses on local, short-term implementation.*

Mechanisms for achieving closer working could include service level agreements based on long-term evaluation and knowledge management needs. In theory, this should be easier to do now through the public health networks. The recent *Choosing Health* white paper recognises many of these issues, particularly the need for a strategy and to build capacity.[13] It further identifies lack of co-ordination between funders, lack of investment in behavioural change, and lack of investigation into what will reduce inequalities.

In response, the white paper proposes a range of initiatives including review of the current strategy, new initiatives and new funding.[13] Work-force capacity will also be considered as part of the workforce plan, with particular emphasis on strengthening research and evaluation skills among public health specialists and practitioners.

This initiative does, however, only apply to England and focuses on health improvement. There are also academic capacity gaps in the health protection workforce which will need to be addressed, preferably by an overarching approach.

While the white paper does not provide a panacea for all the issues, it does at least raise considerably the profile of academic public health and seek to meet some of the more obvious deficits of recent years. However, sustained efforts will be required to promote the cause of academic public health.

References

1 World Health Organization (1978) *Alma Ata Declaration Primary Health Care*. World Health Organization, Geneva.

2   World Health Organization (1986) *Ottawa Charter for Health Promotion*. World Health Organization, Geneva.

3   Institute of Medicine, Committee for the Study of the Future of Public Health (1988) *The Future of Public Health*. National Academy Press, Washington, DC.

4   Public Health Agency website, www.phac-aspc.gc.ca

5   Department of Health (1988) *Public Health in England. Report of the Committee of Inquiry into the Future Development of the Public Health Function*. Department of Health, London.

6   Winslow CEA (1923) *The Evolution and Significance of the Modern Public Health*. Yale University Press, New York.

7   HM Treasury (2004) *Securing Good Health for the Whole Population – final report*. HM Treasury, London.

8   Whitehead M and Dahlgren G (1991) What can be done about inequalities in health? *Lancet*. **338**: 1059–63.

9   Association of Directors of Public Health (2004) *The Role of the Director of Public Health*. ALPHA, Cambridge.

10 Griffiths S, Wright J and Thorpe A (2005) Public health in transition: views of the specialist workforce. Submitted to *Pub Health Med.*

11 Griffiths S, Jewell T and Donnelly P (2005) Supporting specialist practice: the use of the three domains. *Pub Health Med.* In press.

12 Department of Health (2001) *The CMO's Project to Strengthen the Public Health Function*. Department of Health, London.

13 Perlman F and Gray S (2004) *The Specialist Public Health Workforce in the UK. A Report to the Board of the Faculty of Public Health*. FPH, London.

14 Department of Health (2004) *Choosing Health: making healthy choices easier*. Department of Health, London.

15 Wellcome Trust (2004) *The Challenges and Opportunities for Academic Public Health*. Wellcome Trust, London.

16 www.bma.org.uk/ap.nsf/Content/COMARappendix1 (accessed 8 March 2005).

Developing a modernised and multidisciplinary public health specialist workforce

Chapter 3

Developing a modernised and multidisciplinary public health specialist workforce

Learning points

- A flexible, competency-based approach is needed to develop a well trained workforce at all levels.
- Key drivers include the public health white paper *Choosing Health*, *Modernising Medical Careers*, the UK Voluntary Register and *Agenda for Change*.
- Career pathways and funding streams need to be clarified.
- The Faculty of Public Health has a clear role as the standard-setting body for specialist public health working with other organisations.

History

The Department of Health announced in *Saving Lives: our healthier nation* the creation of a new category of multidisciplinary specialists in public health with equivalent status to their medical consultant colleagues.[1] The official endorsement was followed by *Shifting the Balance of Power* which set out the process for the establishment of primary care trust (PCT)-based public health and ensured that directors of public health (DPH) posts were open to appropriately qualified and experienced people from both medical and non-medical backgrounds.[2]

The Faculty of Public Health (FPH), the specialist standard-setting body, was already making changes in response to Department of Health policy, by opening up examinations to applicants from medical and non-medical backgrounds. In 2002 the FPH agreed that full membership rights should be dependent on acquisition of competencies and qualifications that did not necessarily rely on having a medical degree. This meant that those with relevant public health skills and who met the established standards set could be formally recognised as specialists. The UK Voluntary Register was established in 2003 for the specific purpose of regulating specialists without a formal registering body.[3] This has paved the way for a truly multidisciplinary specialist profession.

Underpinning the development of multidisciplinary specialist practice has been the *principle of equivalence* between medically qualified consultants in public health medicine and specialists from backgrounds other than medicine who reach appropriate levels of competence in specialist public health practice. Assessment of competence has been based on an examination system. The FPH examination process and professional mechanisms, such as advice on job descriptions and appointments processes, were revised on the basis of the equivalence principle and 'Medicine' was dropped from the name of the Faculty.[4,5] In order to be able to register professionals from backgrounds other than medicine working in senior posts in the UK, the Voluntary Register has established a mechanism for accreditation until May 2006 in the first instance, on the basis of retrospective portfolio assessment. The framework for assessment was established through extensive discussions with a variety of professional groups as well as discussion with other countries. Specialists accredited onto the voluntary register will be required to undergo revalidation including meeting the requirements for continuing professional development (CPD) in exactly the same way as doctors on the General Medical Council (GMC) register, to ensure maintenance of standards.

Specialist training

Multidisciplinary training programmes have now been established in all regions of England. Figure 3.1 illustrates the training pathway.

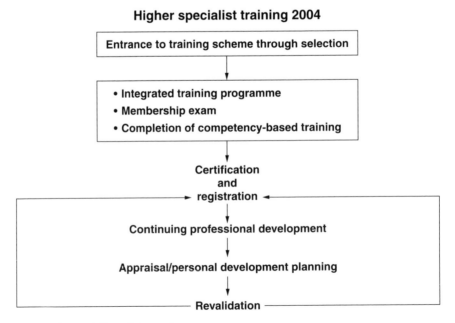

Figure 3.1: The specialist training pathway.

Currently, a specialist training programme will provide the opportunity to take Part I and Part II of the Faculty's exams (currently under review) – which demonstrate the 'know how' of specialist practice. In addition the formal training programmes are based on the acquisition of competencies – the 'show how' – which need to be acquired to be registered as a specialist. These are formally assessed within the postgraduate deanery structures, now working closely with workforce development directorates, who have responsibility for funding and developing specialist public health careers across the professions. All those who enrol are expected to achieve common recognised and validated standards of professional practice.

Framework for training

The underlying themes that underpin training and professional practice are:

- an emphasis on competency-based frameworks
- flexible approaches for training at all levels
- continual lifelong learning with appraisal and certification
- registration to provide public protection.

The competency framework for training is based on the ten key areas of specialist practice which were derived in consultation with a wide variety of specialists and agreed with the four Chief Medical Officers (CMOs) in England, Scotland, Wales and Northern Ireland in June 2002 (*see* Box 3.1).[6]

Box 3.1: The ten key areas of specialist practice[6]

1 Surveillance and assessment of the population's health and wellbeing.
2 Promoting and protecting the population's health and wellbeing.
3 Developing quality and risk management within an evaluative culture.
4 Collaborative working for health.
5 Developing health programmes and services and reducing inequalities.
6 Policy and strategy development and implementation.
7 Working with and for communities.
8 Strategic leadership for health.
9 Research and development.
10 Ethically managing self, people and resources.

These ten key areas form the basis for professional standards. They provide a comprehensive framework for generic public health competencies, including for use at practitioner level.[7]

They are complemented by professional expectations laid out in *Good Public Health Practice*, based on the GMC's *Good Medical Practice*.[8,9] *Good Public Health Practice* forms the basis for appraisal, underpinning CPD, and for revalidation. The headings under which good public health practice appraisal is assessed are:

- good public health practice
- maintaining good public health practice
- teaching and training
- relations with individuals and communities
- working with colleagues
- probity
- health.

Further detail is given on these areas on the FPH website. *Good Public Health Practice* provides the framework for annual appraisal and personal development planning which will, in time, contribute to revalidation. Work is currently underway to make explicit the expectation of standards in practice as well as clarifying the processes around them.

Registration

Before the development of the Voluntary Register, only doctors could be registered as public health specialists, and then only with the GMC. The process of registration relied on certification of fitness to practise. Registration was usually via the Specialist Training Authority on completion of a formal training programme. Exceptions to this route were for those coming from other countries. In either circumstance there was an assumption that specialist standards as set out by the royal colleges/ faculties had been met. This process is now under the auspices of the Postgraduate Medical Education Board. With the development of multi-disciplinary public health there were several changes in registration processes. The most significant was the establishment of the Voluntary Register for those without a professional register. In addition, as a result of discussions with the Council for Health Care Regulators (now called the Council for Healthcare Regulatory Excellence (CHRE)) and other professional registering bodies, the notion of equivalence was extended between registers. The General Dental Council (GDC) agreed specialist public health standards for consultants in dental public health which were equivalent to those for doctors on the GMC and for the Voluntary Register. Discussion along these lines have also taken place with the Nursing and Midwifery Council (NMC) and the Royal Pharmaceutical Society of Great

Britain, the outcome of which will be determined through further consultation. At the time of going to press, there are reviews of the GMC and other professional regulatory bodies.

Taking the workforce to the next stage: moving to a competency-based approach

The challenge faced in widening specialist practice to its multidisciplinary base was to make explicit expected standards and to establish mechanisms that ensured they were maintained. This required developing a broader and acceptable definition of specialist practice which recognised the valuable contribution to be made by a wide range of experts previously outside the professional framework. The concept of defined specialists who would be expected to have competence to a certain level across the framework of practice but would be 'expert' within certain areas has been proposed. Work is currently underway, funded by the UK Departments of Health, to develop and consult on specific defined competency frameworks. Interested groups include public health intelligence specialists, health promotion specialists, health psychologists, public health pharmacists and nutritionists, environmental health and health protection staff, academics and health economists, all from backgrounds other than medicine. Again, they would have equivalent status to the generalist specialists.

At the heart of making a success of this remains the notion of equivalence: it is essential that the requirements to be met by the different types of specialist are defined in a transparent and robust way as being of equal weight and value. It is clear also that equivalence needs to be established between prospective and retrospective routes to attaining specialist accreditation. The equivalence of these processes must be accepted as such by the broad public health church. The FPH is also exploring ways to develop public health specialisms as possible alternative routes for higher specialist training in public health.

Linked to changes such as those outlined in *Modernising Medical Careers*, which is radically changing medical training,[11] the philosophy behind the concept of 'defined specialist' could offer exciting possibilities including rebuilding links to other clinical disciplines and introducing careers that combine clinical practice and public health competencies in practice.

Modernising Medical Careers promotes new competency-based pathways for doctors.[11] It provides the opportunity for new careers to emerge whereby doctors in training can remain in their chosen specialties and acquire competencies in other disciplines. This is particularly relevant for public health, for example where community paediatricians, or general practitioners (GPs) may wish to acquire public health competencies, and public health specialists may wish to retain clinical skills.

For specialists from backgrounds other than medicine the national *Agenda for Change* programme through its *Knowledge and Skills Framework* will also provide opportunities.[12,13] In common with *Modernising Medical Careers*, it embraces the notion of career development through competency progression. Over time there will be a clear choice of career paths for public health which will have the competencies defined and mapped against practitioner and specialist standards and professional qualifications. This will create opportunities for practitioners to move to specialist levels through competency acquisition. It will also offer new career opportunities within public health.

Further work will be needed in due course to map public health competencies across other registering bodies such as the GMC and NMC, in the same way as has been possible to register consultants in dental public health with the GDC.

This all suggests that a new and more flexible model of training in public health is needed, which can take people from an interest in public health, through practitioner to specialist level within both generalist and defined specialties. These opportunities underline the need for the public health workforce development plan required by *Choosing Health*,[14] and for greater clarity on career pathways and funding streams for training.

> *The workforce plan for public health will need to take account of the complex mix of expertise required and of the need to develop capacity of public health practitioners as well as public health specialists.*[15]

Thus this will meet the criticism of Wanless, who stressed the importance of strategic workforce planning in public health.[15]

One of the other challenges will be to reconcile the planning divide between medicine and other professionals maintained through Department of Health policies and funding streams, which have, to date, failed to develop frameworks that bring the professions together in a way supportive of the avowed principles of multidisciplinary training for all healthcare workers. This could be achieved by building on existing frameworks, e.g. as shown in the representation of higher specialist training (*see* Figure 3.1), and integrating public health into mainstream workforce development in the NHS.

Achieving the objective of multisectoral education – for example with local government – still poses problems, particularly of resources. Nevertheless, many of the building blocks are now in place to allow public health to move forward as a truly multidisciplinary profession.

References

1 Department of Health (1999) *Saving Lives: our healthier nation*. Department of Health, London.

2 Department of Health (2001) *Shifting the Balance of Power in England*. Department of Health, London.
3 www.publichealthregister.org.uk (accessed 9 March 2005).
4 Faculty of Public Health (2002) *Guidance for the Appointment of Specialists in Public Health*. FPH, London.
5 Faculty of Public Health (2003) *About the Faculty*. www.fph.org.uk (accessed 28 April 2005).
6 Faculty of Public Health. www.fph.org.uk (accessed 9 March 2005).
7 Health Scotland (2004) *Occupational Standards/Competencies for Public Health Practice. A joint report*. Health Scotland, Edinburgh.
8 Faculty of Public Health (2001) *Good Public Health Practice, Standards for Public Health Practice*. FPH, London.
9 General Medical Council (1995) *Maintaining Good Medical Practice*. www.gmc-uk.org/standards/mgmp.htm (accessed 9 March 2005).
10 www.fph.org.uk (accessed 9 March 2005).
11 Department of Health (2004) *Modernising Medical Careers: the next steps. The future shape of foundation, specialist and general practice training programmes*. Department of Health, London.
12 Department of Health (2004) *Agenda for Change: final agreement*. Department of Health, London.
13 Department of Health (2004) *NHS Knowledge and Skills Framework and Development Review Guidance*. Department of Health, London.
14 Department of Health (2004) *Choosing Health: making healthy choices easier*. Department of Health, London.
15 HM Treasury (2004) *Securing Good Health for the Whole Population*. HM Treasury, London.

Public health specialist practice in community settings: primary care and local government

Public health specialist practice in community settings: primary care and local government

Learning points

- Public health specialists play a key role within primary care and local government.
- Existing powers and opportunities can be used as levers to engage local government, e.g. scrutiny, local strategic partnerships, powers, director of public health (DPH) appointments, DPH annual reports.
- The tension between the corporate and public health agendas for DPHs should be recognised.
- Greater capacity at primary care trust (PCT) level is needed to enable DPHs to serve their communities more effectively, so that they in turn can support other health professionals including staff within local government and primary care in making prevention and health improvement part of their daily work.
- The full integration of public health programmes into joint performance management with common performance measures developed for primary care and local government will raise the profile of public health in statutory organisations.
- Co-terminosity with population boundaries facilitates joint working between local government and public health.
- Support to commissioning is re-emerging as a key role for public health.
- Other specialists have key roles to play within community settings.

Setting a context: evolving relationships

Public health is not the prerogative of the NHS, or indeed any single part of the public sector. It is an intrinsic part of the mainstream activities of both the statutory and non-statutory sectors. . . . The key role of local government in tackling health inequalities and supporting the development of the fully engaged scenario needs proper recognition and support (p. 2).[1]

Evolving relationships: primary care

Traditionally, the focus of primary care has been on the care of individual patients, with population health the prerogative of public health professionals. In 1978 this distinction was challenged by the *Declaration of Alma Ata*, which suggested that:

primary health care reflects and evolves from the economic conditions and sociocultural and political characteristics of the country and its communities and is based on the application of the relevant results of social, biomedical and health services research and public health experience (point VII.1).[2]

Distinguishing between primary medical care and primary healthcare, this document advocated a people-centred multi- and intersectoral approach to healthcare. The principles of primary healthcare have the potential to create a new culture in health services globally, with, as Barnard suggests:

the ultimate promise . . . of 'seamless' community health development embracing its different dimensions of medical and social care and the various forms of protection and support offered to the community.[3]

As the *Ljubljana Charter on Reforming Health Care*, 1996, stated:

health care should first and foremost lead to better health and quality of life for people. . . . Reforms with primary health care as a philosophy should ensure that health services at all levels protect and promote health, improve the quality of life, prevent and treat diseases. . . . There is a need to develop a set of managerial functions and public health infrastructures entrusted with the tasks of guiding or influencing the overall system to achieve the desired improvements in the population's health.[4]

The interrelationship between public health and primary healthcare could not be more explicit. The vision, the goal and the infrastructure are mutually supportive. Community engagement, particularly between primary healthcare and local government, is integral to achieving this goal – a goal which has been paraphrased by Wanless as 'the fully engaged scenario'.[5] This chapter will reflect on the role of public health specialists in taking this forward by facilitating cross-sectoral engagement.

While the two paradigms of individual patients and population focus have often been juxtaposed, during the 1990s the organisational changes in the NHS drew public health and primary care professionals more closely together, particularly with the creation first of primary care groups (PCGs) and then of PCTs with responsibility for improving the health of their populations. Within the context of these changes the Faculty of Public Health (Medicine) (FPH) and the National Public Health and Primary Care Group conducted a survey of all 100 health authority DPHs in England in 1998 to explore how they saw their contribution. Their response highlighted a focus of activities which included: information analyses, health needs assessments, reviewing the evidence base and effectiveness of services and procedures, health promotion activities and developing guidelines.[6]

In 2000 the Faculty of Public Health Medicine, as part of its submission to the House of Commons Select Committee on Public Health, produced a framework for developing public health in primary care which described public health functions that could be delivered within a PCT and those which would need to span a larger population base.[7] This framework identified the need for local primary care staff with relevant skills to deliver the new roles that were required as a result of this reorganisation of services, as well as the need for training and development opportunities. The framework also highlighted the crucial need for joint work not only with local government but between public health academics and service colleagues to support these new organisations. The importance of public health leadership to co-ordinate new arrangements across a complex and wide range of partners was also emphasised.

The advantages of closer working between general practice and public health have been drawn out in a series of reports which highlighted the need to create better and closer ways of working, as well as the key contribution that general practice can make to important public health goals.[8-11] The emphasis in policy documents has continued to grow, with population approaches to improving health and preventing disease achieving higher profile. The Wanless report in 2002, which presents an economic case for health improvement puts the case for public health in stark relief.[5]

The desirable health outcomes depicted in the fully engaged scenario are only likely to come about with a step change in the way public health is viewed, resourced and delivered nationally.

More recently Royal College of General Practitioners (RCGP) has re-emphasised the role of general practitioners (GPs) in public health.[12] As the organisation of primary care continues to change with the implementation of the new contracts, the focus on patient- (individual-) centred care, more engagement in commissioning, and expectation of new relationships as a consequence of new structures such as children's trusts and plurality of providers including foundation trusts, the specialist profession faces new challenges.

Evolving relationships: with local government

Until 1974, public health services were part of local government. Local authorities retain, in the services they deliver, a large impact on many of the determinants of health, for example through their roles in:

- education
- social services
- housing
- environment, transport and planning
- leisure and recreation
- crime, protective services and community safety
- waste and recycling.[13]

The historical links between public health specialists and local government had been weakened by the focus on health services management during the 1980s and early 1990s. However, Acheson's review of the public health function acted as a trigger to reinvigorate engagement with the broader determinants of health and the local government links.[11]

A survey of two health authority areas around this time identified:[14]

- **a wide spectrum of views on what public health is and the differing contributions organisations can make**: local government, community health council, primary and community service leaders perceived public health as tackling the broader social, environmental and economic determinants of health. However, health authorities and hospital trusts considered the public health role fell within the remit of the healthcare system, with the public health departments helping with commissioning, prioritisation, clinical effectiveness, performance management and information gathering within the NHS
- **great importance attached to partnership working**: general enthusiasm by all organisations for working together to improve health, but emphasising the need for senior commitment to developing a common agenda.

The survey also identified the need for:

- **supra-PCT public health expertise**: certain statutory public health functions, i.e. communicable disease and specialist commissioning would be better provided through networks covering larger populations sharing available skills
- **specialist public health input**: creative ways of sharing capacity
- **raising awareness of the public health role of PCTs**: the PCT workforce needed to be involved in public health programmes, working with specialist support
- **public health skills of primary care practitioners**: these need to be nurtured and developed
- **common agendas with local government**.

A further report on taking forward ideas to strengthen joint working between health authorities and local authorities on the broader public health agenda identified a number of key factors for successful joint working.[15] These included working with elected members of local authorities, often very interested in health issues and strong advocates for public health, crucial in getting key messages over to members of the public. One of the blocks identified was the difficulty in sharing information, for example in establishing local profiles, and another difficulty was how to find ways of breaking down barriers to sharing funding. Options for encouraging better joint working included joint posts, and shared training opportunities. The DPH annual report could be formally reported to local authorities.

The report by the Public Health Resource Unit (PHRU) on promoting healthy partnerships looked at how the factors affecting health (*see* Table 4.1) could be used to identify areas of synergy between organisational agendas.[16,17]

Table 4.1: Factors affecting health (source: Department of Health, 1998).[17]

Fixed	*Social and economic*	*Environment*	*Lifestyle*	*Access to services*
Genes	Poverty	Air quality	Diet	Education
Sex	Employment	Housing	Physical activity	NHS
Ageing	Social exclusion	Water quality	Smoking	Social services
		Social environment	Alcohol	Transport
			Sexual behaviour	Leisure
			Drugs	

The identification of vulnerable groups in the population for which the organisations share a common responsibility can provide a common ground for partnership working. By focusing on the needs of the vulnerable groups in the population which fall within the responsibilities of local government, the health service, the voluntary sector and other public sector agencies, a significant commonality of interest can be identified, and a partnership agenda with shared outcomes generated. Such an approach is relevant to making local strategic partnerships (LSPs) a tool for promoting public health.

The PHRU report, using the work of Mitchell (*see* Box 4.1), suggested that this approach could enable agencies to share good practice and learning, to complement the skills and experience of others and undertake joint consultation work with communities and the local population, and possibly provide a basis for strategic planning.[16,18]

Box 4.1: Vulnerable groups in the population which provide a common ground for partnership (source: Mitchell, 1997)[18]

- The elderly
- Children and families, including lone parent families, teenage pregnancies
- Those who have a mental illness
- Those who have a learning disability
- Those who have physical and/or sensory impairments
- Those who have problems from drug and/or alcohol abuse
- Those who have HIV/AIDS
- Patients who require palliative care

Moving forward: setting up PCTs

When *Shifting the Balance of Power*, was implemented on April 1 2002,[19] health structures went overnight from 100 health authorities to some 350 PCTs and 28 strategic health authorities (SHAs), shifting the role of primary care organisations from delivery of specific programmes to an explicit responsibility not only for healthcare, but also for the health of populations:

> *PCTs will be responsible for assessing the health needs of their local community and preparing plans for health improvement which recognise the diversity of health needs. A strengthened public health function will be needed in PCTs to support this needs assessment and to ensure that public health surveillance and population screening are carried out across local communities (p. 13).*

The dissolution of district health authorities and the move to PCGs, (encompassing populations of around 100 000) and PCTs (encompassing populations around 150 000 or more) at the beginning of this century brought public health consultants and specialists into a much closer relationship with primary care and local government. Three key public health roles for PCTs were identified:

- improving the health of the community through health needs assessment, plans for improvement, LSPs and 'a significantly strengthened public health function'
- securing the provision of medical, nursing, dental, pharmacy and optical services throughout their area
- integrating health and social care by working with local authorities.[19]

The local public health function was to be led by the DPH (a board level requirement for each PCT), supported by a dedicated team of consultants/ specialist staff, health promotion specialists and health information analysts.

In his seminal address to the Faculty of Public Health, Lord Hunt outlined the expectation for the DPHs, saying they will:

> *focus their activity on local neighbourhoods and communities leading and driving programmes to improve health and reduce inequalities – they will not be a remote, strategic figure – he or she will be well known, respected and credible with local people – particularly those in the most deprived communities, local authorities, general practitioners and other local clinicians.*[20]

The DPH was established as a leadership role, providing public health advice to the PCT board and management team, leading the delivery of public health programmes and engaging and working with primary and community care professionals and local government and local authority staff to meet PCT targets. The professional role of the DPH was developed to reflect activity and responsibility within the framework of the ten key areas of practice.[21]

Table 4.2 sets out the main tasks of the PCT public health specialist workforce mapped against these ten key areas of public health.

Many if not all of these functions can only be delivered in partnership with colleagues in primary care or local government.

Developing relationships and opportunities in primary care

With the increasing emphasis on chronic disease management, the engagement of primary care clinicians not only in primary prevention but in secondary prevention has become increasingly important. An FPH/ RCGP paper in 2001 looked at ways in which primary care clinicians could actively contribute to the public health agenda.[22] Analysis of effective delivery of specific National Service Framework (NSF) programmes such as coronary heart disease and diabetes, of screening programmes, of advice on lifestyle factors, of mental healthcare and of care of older people highlighted the need to build up public health skills within the primary care workforce. The immediate focus for joint working needed to be on the delivery of programmes and meeting public health targets. The new GP contract, and its *Quality and Outcomes Framework*, provides opportunities and levers to set and deliver public health targets through clinical practice.[23]

Table 4.2: PCT public health specialist workforce.

Key area	Examples of tasks
Surveillance, assessment of population health	• Lead and co-ordinate the assessment of health needs and inequalities • Identify areas for action within the local population • Establish systems for health surveillance • Monitor local basket of health inequalities indicators • Lead health equity audits • Produce an annual report
Promoting and protecting population's health and wellbeing	• Responsibility for provision of screening programmes for the local population and meeting targets for screening and immunisation/vaccination programmes • Lead the contribution of the PCT to effective local arrangements to support surveillance and control of health protection and environmental control • Develop/lead health improvement initiatives and strategies
Developing quality and risk within an evaluative culture	• Develop effective clinical governance systems • Support development of evidence-based practice within multiprofessional teams, the evaluation of the effectiveness of healthcare provision and programmes and the development of appropriate health outcome measures • Input to primary, secondary and specialist care commissioning
Developing health programmes and services and reducing inequalities	• Establish local targets and consider the impact of national targets for the improvement of health and the reduction of inequalities and timely access to high-quality health services • Contribute public health leadership to the commissioning process
Policy and strategy development and implementation	• Develop local health strategy including advising on effective evidence-based healthcare delivery
Strategic leadership for health	• Lead the PCT's contribution to building partnerships to ensure the widest possible participation in the health and healthcare agenda
Working with and for communities	• Take a leadership role with local communities in helping them to take action to tackle long-standing and widening health inequalities issues
Research and development	• Work with information managers in the PCT and local authority to develop the information base
Ethically managing self, people and resources (including education and continuing professional development (CPD))	• Effective leadership of the public health team, including management and staff development

While the positive policy shift is welcome, the higher profile of public health in primary care is challenging for specialists. The current trend in primary care is moving full circle, with the move of GPs to the helm of primary and secondary care commissioning:

> the new proposals bear striking similarities to fundholding, sharing such characteristics as budget holding by general practices and direct financial incentive for general practitioners.[24]

The challenge for DPHs now is to reconsider how best their skills in health needs assessment, information analysis and reviewing effectiveness can support GP primary and secondary care commissioning, as well as how to tackle the developing health improvement agenda with its focus not only on including health education within clinical interactions, but on engaging all sectors of the community in health improvement. As Wanless has pointed out:

> difficulties remain in some areas due to capacity problems, the impact of recent organisational changes and the lack of alignment of performance management mechanisms between partners.[5]

The full benefits of public health engagement in primary care therefore requires greater capacity and capability than exists at present. The demand for public health skills at all levels not only of the NHS workforce but across other sectors including local government, has increased to unprecedented levels. Public health specialists, GPs, community nurses and primary care teams all have a role to play in improving health and reducing health inequalities. The contribution from other practitioners, including pharmacists, is growing in prominence.

Developing relationships and opportunities with local government

As the joint response from the FPH and the Local Government Association, to the Wanless Consultation in 2003, stated:

> Public health is not the prerogative of the NHS, or indeed any single part of the public sector. It is an intrinsic part of the mainstream activities of both the statutory and non-statutory sectors. . . . The key role of local government in tackling health inequalities and supporting the development of the fully engaged scenario needs proper recognition and support. (p. 2).[25]

Inequalities in health continue to exist – if not to grow.[26] Deprived communities experience higher rates of morbidity and mortality. Joint working is essential to address these inequalities. At a local level, the challenge is to work with local government, the voluntary sector, local businesses and employers.[27] Public health specialists need to facilitate this process. But there are also challenges to the NHS to use the changes of recent reforms to develop the public health function, empower public health teams, and engage and motivate the NHS workforce.

The Wanless report, the *Choosing Health* consultation and *Choosing Health* itself offer an opportunity to review and rethink the specialist role, including the relationship between local authorities and the public health service, to build on the synergies which will allow closer working with communities and provide the opportunities for better health for all, but particularly the most disadvantaged.[5,28,29]

Joint appointments

One of the key changes post-*Shifting the Balance of Power*[19] has been to create joint appointments between PCTs and local councils of posts including that of the DPH. There is an increasing move towards joint plans and shared targets with creative use of council powers and scrutiny processes. This has been emphasised within *Choosing Health*.[29]

The most successful joint appointments, according to the Office for Public Management's (OPM's) research, were those where partner organisations had a clear strategic framework, and clarity of what the appointment could and could not be expected to achieve. The added value of the joint post is to achieve real and effective partnership, with the leadership skills and personal qualities of the individual in the post being of prime importance to ensure effective delivery (*see* Box 4.2).

Box 4.2: Joint appointments: critical success factors (source: OPM, 2001)[30]

- Early planning
- Clear strategic purpose
- Funding
- Recruitment
- Administrative and logistical support
- Induction
- Performance management
- Training, development and personal support
- A systematic process for strategic review
- A process for influencing partner agendas
- Formative reflection and evaluation

For public health, where working across organisational boundaries can add extra complexity into an already over-extended specialist public health service, these factors are particularly important. To quote from the *Choosing Health* survey responses:

> *[joint appointments] may work well with single tier local authorities (e.g. unitaries) but create significant issues where there is both county and district level. We should focus more public health attention on delivering effective programmes with partners.*[31]

There are many good examples of positive outcomes from joint working between local government and primary care in which public health specialists play a key role. One of the features these experiences tend to share is working in a PCT which shares a common population and common boundary with their local authority. In addition a DPH with a passion for the shared agenda can effectively facilitate the complex process of partnership working. However, there is considerable variability across the country in local government structures, and lack of co-terminosity with PCTs in many parts of the country, especially where county and district councils are in place, mitigating against effective joint working. The capacity seminars in 2004 demonstrated that where PCTs are not co-terminous with councils there are enormous complexities in delivering the broader public health agenda especially where support teams are small.[32]

  The *Choosing Health* survey found that 79% of the respondents saw co-terminosity as a key goal to facilitating partnership working because it facilitates joint working, and makes planning and relationships easier.[31] Other observations included that many workers in different organisations are engaged in programmes that have a public health impact, but often the links are not made between those working on similar agendas, thereby inhibiting the efficacy and sustainability of these programmes. Another reflection was that although pump priming programmes are useful, sustainability and mainstream delivery are essential components of ad-dressing the public health agenda in the long term. As one DPH responded to the *Choosing Health* survey:

> *This [mainstream funding] is the only way to deliver Wanless's aspirations. Otherwise forget the fully engaged scenario, forget solid progress, and expect an ever increasing proportion of GDP [gross domestic product] being required for the National Sickness Service just to stand still.*[31]

Co-terminosity and joint appointments may be 'the ideal way' to deliver improved health for the population, with public health specialists working across all relevant organisations to achieve horizontal integration – but they are not the only way. Integration is 'a matter of degree, not an end state'.[33] There are three possible routes to achieving effective integration:

1 signposting and co-ordination
2 managed processes
3 integrated organisations.

The LSP provides one example of how integration can work (*see* Chapter 7).

Common assessment: joint targets

Competing interests between health and local authorities may mean that many public health opportunities are overlooked. Also, the need to 'balance the books' while delivering on the 'must-dos' creates a tension within the NHS, often undermining the willingness to be involved in public health initiatives. Joint targets are an option to create legitimacy for joint working. Examples of national targets include:

* to improve access to services: increase the participation of problem drug users in drug treatment programmes by 100% by 2008 and increase year on year the proportion of users successfully sustaining or completing treatment programmes.

The benefits of joint targets include their ability to:

* help align objectives
* help with public service agreements (PSAs)
* strengthen horizontal integration.

Following *Choosing Health* there is greater emphasis on public health in the cross-government public service agreements, particularly those for smoking, obesity, sexual health, inequalities and workforce development (*see* Box 4.3).

Box 4.3: Public service agreements[34]

PSAs set out each department's aims, objectives and key outcome-based targets. The targets measure changes in the level of quality of a specific service, or an improvement in the lives of people across the UK. There are around 130 PSA targets across all the government departments – an average of fewer than seven per department. The Department of Health's target page suggests it has 12 targets to meet, with the Secretary of State responsible for delivery of the targets.

Additional health-related targets can be found in other departmental PSAs, however, for instance the target for SureStart is the responsibility of the Department of Education and Skills. These targets set an agenda for action for public health, providing a tool to mainstream public health projects within both health and local government, with a key role for SHAs in monitoring delivery against the targets.

The reduced number of national targets creates more headroom for PCTs to set local targets in response to local needs and priorities. These will need to be agreed with local authorities and other partner organisations (*see* Box 4.4).

Box 4.4: Principles for local target setting

In developing local plans PCTs should ensure they:
- are in line with population needs
- address local service gaps
- deliver equity
- are evidence based
- are developed in partnership with other NHS bodies and the local authorities
- offer value for money.[35]

In the *Choosing Health* consultation exercise with specialists, joint targets were strongly supported but the specialists were concerned to have the right targets and not necessarily more targets.

The new Planning and Priorities Framework reduces the number of national targets and will allow PCTs with local authorities to set some local targets (*see* Chapter 7). The inclusion of public health in the Healthcare Commission framework for reviewing organisational delivery was also a welcome development, especially given the encouraging suggestion of joint reviews with the Audit Commission for PCTs and local authorities across shared geographical boundaries. This will increase the emphasis on and degree of integration of public health programmes, and was strongly supported by specialists who welcome the inclusion of public health in national performance management systems. They supported a greater presence in the balanced score card system of performance management of PCTs as an example of the advantage to be gained through mainstreaming public health and public health issues, thereby enhancing profile and delivery.

> If public health targets were 'hanging offences' they would be given much higher priority.[31]

However, capacity deficits mean that imaginative ways are needed to ensure delivery. In some places, mergers of specialist support teams between PCTs have taken place with more training and engagement of local practitioners from primary care and community services such as pharmacy and dentistry.

> We need more people with some public health training and skills delivering practical public health programmes.[31]

References

1 Faculty of Public Health, NHS Confederation, Local Government Association, UK Public Health Association, Association of Public Health Observatories (2003) *Joint Response to Securing Good Health for the Whole Population.* www.lga.gov.uk/download.asp?path=/Documents/Briefing/Our_Work/social%20affairs/Jointsubmission.pdf (accessed 9 March 2005).

2 World Health Organization (1978) *The Declaration of Alma Ata.* World Health Organization, Geneva.

3 Barnard K, Norrby K and Philalithis T (1999) *Tipping the Balance Towards a Healthier Health Care.* www.phcttb.org (accessed 9 March 2005).

4 World Health Organization (1996) *The Ljubljana Charter on Reforming Health Care.* www.euro.who.int/AboutWHO/Policy/20010927_5 (accessed 9 March 2005).

5 HM Treasury (2002) *Securing Our Future: taking a long term view.* HM Treasury, London.

6 FPH survey (1998) Unpublished.

7 FPH response (2000) Unpublished.

8 Department of Health (2001) *The Report of the CMO's Project to Strengthen the Public Health Function.* Department of Health, London.

9 House of Commons Select Committee (2001) *Second Report: public health-1* (session 2000-1): HC30-1.

10 All Party Parliamentary Group on Primary Care (2001) *Primary Care Trusts: can they deliver on public health?* HMSO, London.

11 Department of Health (1998) *Independent Inquiry into Inequalities in Health, Chair: Sir Donald Acheson.* HMSO, London.

12 Royal College of General Practitioners (2004) *The Future of General Practice: A Statement by the RCGP.* Royal College of General Practitioners, London.

13 Local Authorities' Gateway to National Support. www.local.gov.uk/ (accessed 9 March 2005).

14 Griffiths S, Wright J and Grice D (2001) Public health: a tale of two counties. *Health Serv J.* 111: 30–1.

15 Select Committee (2000) *Inquiry into Public Health.* www.parliament.uk/commons/selcom01/hltpnt13.htm (accessed 9 March 2005).

16 Public Health Resource Unit (1998) *Partnership Working on the Broader Public Health Agenda.* Public Health Resource Unit, Oxford.

17 Department of Health (1998) *Our Healthier Nation: a contract for health.* The Stationery Office, London.

18 Mitchell G (1997) *Towards a Strategic Relationship Between Unitary Authorities and Berkshire Health Authority, a Potential Shared Agenda.* Cited in PHRU (1998), p.33.

19 Department of Health (2001) *Shifting the Balance of Power.* Department of Health, London.

20 Parliamentary Under Secretary of State for Health (2001) *First Annual Faculty of Public Health Lecture,* delivered by Lord Hunt, November 2001.

21 Association of Directors of Public Health. *The Role of the Director of Public Health.* www.alpha.nhs.uk/Conferences/ConfArchive/AssDPH%20March04/DPH%20Leaflet.pdf (accessed 9 March 2005).

22 Royal College of General Practitioners/Faculty of Public Health Medicine (2001) *Public Health in the New NHS Structures: the primary care perspective.* Royal College of General Practitioners/Faculty of Public Health Medicine, London.

23 Department of Health (2003) *Delivery Investment in General Practice. Implementing the New GMS Contract.* Department of Health, London.

24 Lewis RG (2004) Back to the future? [editorial] From 2005 individual general practices can apply to commission services. *BMJ.* **329**: 932.

25 Faculty of Public Health, NHS Confederation, Local Government Association, UK Public Health Association, Association of Public Health Observatories (2003) *Joint Response to Securing Good Health for the Whole Population.* www.lga.gov.uk/download.asp?path=/Documents/Briefing/Our_Work/social%20affairs/Jointsubmission.pdf (accessed 9 March 2005).

26 Department of Health (2003) *Tackling Inequalities in Health: an action plan.* Department of Health, London.

27 Department of Health (2001) *Shifting the Balance of Power: securing delivery.* Department of Health, London.

28 Department of Health (2004) *Choosing Health?* White Paper Consultation. Department of Health, London.

29 Department of Health (2004) *Choosing Health: making healthy choices easier.* Department of Health, London.

30 Office of Public Management (2001) *The Joint Appointments Guide.* Office of Public Management, London.

31 Griffiths S, Wright J and Thorpe A (2005) Public health in transition: views of the specialist workforce. Submitted to *Pub Health Med.*

32 Faculty of Public Health, Public Health Resource Unit and Department of Health (2004) *Joint Workshop Report on Capacity Seminars.* Faculty of Public Health, London. www.fph.org.uk (accessed 29 April 2005).

33 Edwards M and Miller C (2003) *Two, Four, Six, Eight: How we gonna integrate?* Office for Public Management, London.

34 Department of Health (2004) *Annual Report 2004.* www.dh.gov.uk/assetRoot/04/09/83/48/04098348.pdf (accessed 9 March 2005).

35 Department of Health (2004) *National Standards, Local Action.* Department of Health, London.

Health protection

Chapter 5

Health protection

Learning points

There is a need for:

- greater health protection capacity
- clarity about accountability and responsibility for local health protection
- clarity about roles and development of new specialist pathways in agreement with professional bodies, with development of competency-based standards
- continuing professional development in health protection for a wide range of public health specialists with the development of appropriate methods of training including leadership.

Health protection in England has gained greater prominence in recent years. The tragic events of September 11 (9/11) and the need for response to threats of bioterrorism made governments around the world realise that the safety of the public was under increasing threat. In addition, the emergence of new infections, such as severe acute respiratory syndrome (SARS) and the relentless global spread of existing diseases re-emphasise the need to find strategies for their prevention and control. It is clear that the thinking that led the Surgeon General of the US to say in 1969 that 'we can now close the book on infectious disease' was misplaced.[1] One only needs to look at the global burden of disease related to HIV/AIDS, TB and malaria to see that effective response to infections is a priority for public health.

The lessons from the SARS epidemic serve to highlight both the universal challenge of controlling infections and the common lessons learnt for organisation of specialist services. In the review of the experiences in Hong Kong and Canada it became obvious that specialist capacity was stretched and inadequate, ways of working across communities especially between hospitals and primary care were inadequate, that communication was poor and control of infection procedures inadequate.[2]

Box 5.1: The SARS epidemic: skills required

The SARS epidemic which began in Southern China, spread to Hong Kong in early March with the outbreak of atypical pneumonia among healthcare workers in the large teaching hospital. Hong Kong officials only became aware of the outbreak of atypical pneumonia which had infected a high number of healthcare workers several months after it had taken a grip in Guangdong, this despite 300 000 people crossing the border each day. Such a delay high-lighted the need for *surveillance systems and communication*.

The epidemic in healthcare workers emphasised the need for preparedness to respond to emergencies, robust *control of infection policies, plans and procedures* as well as the need for *surge capacity*. Some of the confusion between what was a hospital and what was a community case made it clear that a *population-based approach* was needed, supported by good information links in future epidemics to make sure gaps in responses, particularly contact tracing, did not occur. The positive response by the clinical community showed how essential *clinicians, supported by academic colleagues*, are to handling an epidemic. The importance of understanding *environmental determinants* and their impact on disease was also critical to the public health decisions being made. The key lessons learnt from this experience were the need for *good relationships with the community* and the key role of the *media*.

The experience of SARS spells out the challenges specialists face as well as the systems needed to underpin their practice. Effective response to future threats will require the gaps identified to be filled not only in countries hit by SARS but elsewhere as well (*see* Box 5.1).[3]

The response to the increasing need for health protection in England was the Chief Medical Officer's (CMO's) strategy *Getting Ahead of the Curve*.[4] This redefined health protection (HP), linking together the need for response to infectious disease and chemical and radiation hazards with that to threats from bioterrorism and emergencies. The Health Protection Agency (HPA) was created as the authoritative body, a key part of the public health service to take an overview of these areas.

Its creation brought together a group of existing organisations:

- The Public Health Laboratory Service, including the Communicable Disease Surveillance Centre and Central Public Health Laboratory
- The Centre for Applied Microbiology and Research
- The National Focus for Chemical Incidents
- the regional service provider units that support the management of chemical incidents

- The National Poisons Information Service
- NHS public health staff responsible for infectious disease control, emergency planning, and other protection support.

The National Radiological Protection Board became part of the organisation in April 2005.

Initially a special health authority, from April 2005 the HPA will work closely with but be independent of the NHS as a non-departmental public body.

The vision statement from the HPA states that:

> our aim is to protect health, prevent harm and prepare for threats, providing leadership and advocacy, enabling communities and individuals to protect their health, working with partners, locally, nationally and internationally, bringing the best science and specialist skills.[5]

Its main areas of concern are:

- to advise government on public health protection policies and programmes
- to deliver services and to support the NHS and other agencies in protecting people from infections, poisons, chemical and radiation hazards
- to provide an impartial and authoritative source of information and advice to professionals and the public
- to respond to new threats to public health and to provide a rapid response to health protection emergencies
- to improve knowledge about health protection through research and development, education and training.[5]

The work of the HPA falls mainly under four areas:

1 local and regional services (LARS) which provides local response to outbreaks of infection, chemical incidents and emergencies
2 work on infections via specialist and reference laboratories (Centre for Infections)
3 environmental work, providing scientific and medical advice to the NHS and other bodies (Centre for Radiation, Chemical and Environmental Hazards)
4 emergency preparedness and response to ensure preparedness for major emergencies (Centre for Emergency Preparedness and Response).

Priority areas of work include programmes to reduce the incidence and consequences of sexually transmitted diseases, gastrointestinal infections, healthcare-associated infection including methicillin-resistant *Staphylococcus aureus* (MRSA), hepatitis B and C and vaccine preventable diseases. There are also programmes to improve protection against the adverse effects of exposure to ionising and non-ionising radiation as well as the adverse health risks of acute and chronic exposure to chemicals and poisons.

Who are the public health specialists in the HPA and who do they work with?

The creation of the HPA has led to the redefinition of what is meant by specialist practice in public health in health protection, drawing together expertise and services for the areas listed above. The potential links pose new challenges for the development of multidisciplinary practice, extending beyond the borders of the NHS into many other sectors such as environmental and clinical sciences.

The HPA is a major employer of public health specialists. Many of them work within the LARS, which provide local response to outbreaks of infection, chemical incidents and emergencies. These specialists may well have been consultants in communicable diseases within the NHS health authorities prior to organisational change.

Their employment within the HPA has changed relationships both with primary care trusts (PCTs) and professional colleagues in other areas of public health practice.

LARS is currently structured on a regional basis, co-terminous with regional government office boundaries. Its areas of work are:

- investigating and managing incidents and events through:
  - surveillance
  - support to the NHS for service planning and monitoring of health protection services
  - contingency planning
- advising to stakeholders and the public
- contributing to the prevention of communicable diseases and protection from health effects of chemical hazards and radiation
- improving standards by contributing to audit, education and research.

LARS also has the specialist functions of:

- public health microbiology services through a network of laboratories
- information
- emergency planning.

Box 5.2 describes some of the specialists and other public health workforce who work in and with the LARS.

Box 5.2: Health protection professionals: England only[6]

NHS public health staff (mostly in PCTs, but also some in strategic health authorities (SHAs) and trusts)

- Consultants in public health and specialists in public health (including directors of public health (DPHs)) (personal communication, Sue Ibbotson, Regional Director of Health Protection, West Midlands HPA)
- Consultants in public health alone
- Specialists in public health alone
- Public health nurses
- Infection control nurses

HPA LARS general health protection staff

- Consultants in communicable disease control/health protection
- Specialists in health protection
- Health protection nurses (including infection control)

HPA LARS specialised health protection staff (mainly at LARS regional level)

- Environmental health specialists
- Health emergency planning advisers
- Regional epidemiologists
- Epidemiological scientists, information officers

HPA LARS microbiology staff (microbiology, virology, Food Environment Water Laboratory (FEWL))

- Medical microbiologists
- Clinical scientists
- Biomedical scientists
- Medical technical officers
- Assistant technical officers and medical laboratory assistants

Thanks to Rowena Clayton (HPA) for this classification.

The diversity of skills and areas of interest in this group alone demonstrates the challenges in developing a well-trained specialist workforce for health protection. There are, of course, public health specialists in the other parts of the HPA. In particular the national expertise of staff in the Communicable Disease Surveillance Centre (CDSC), who are leading experts in all infectious diseases, are called on not only by local PCTs but also by international colleagues. As such, the CDSC at Colindale provides an invaluable training resource for specialists. Public health specialists are also employed within the other centres across the HPA.

What are the issues for specialist practice?

The creation of the HPA has meant a re-alignment of public health specialist roles. Consultants in Communicable Disease Control (CCDCs) were previously located within district health authority departments of public health, working alongside their generalist public health colleagues. CCDCs and other health protection specialists are now employed within a parallel vertical service to the NHS. Partnership and joint working across organisational boundaries is therefore essential.

Capacity across the country varies, and where there is a good understanding of the relative roles and responsibilities, the system works well. For example, the outbreak of legionnaires' disease in Hereford in 2003 highlighted the close working between all parts of the NHS and HPA in investigating and managing the outbreak. Key messages from the outbreak included the need to be explicit about roles, responsibilities and capabilities in advance of an incident, staying ahead of the media, getting the response structure clear early and handling the politicians.[7]

A further example of the need for close working between the NHS and the HPA lies in detecting an incident and triggering an emergency response. Figure 5.1 highlights the various parties who might be first points of contact.

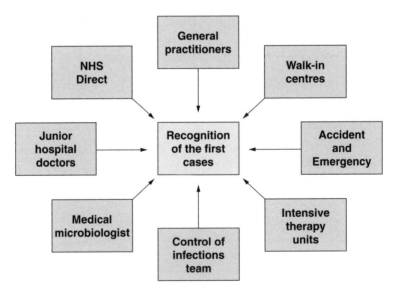

Figure 5.1: Detection of an incident.

Emergency response partners

Specialists in the NHS and in the HPA need to understand their respective roles in detecting and responding to an incident. Developing and maintaining health protection skills in NHS-based specialists remains important not only to provide cover in on-call situations and surge capacity in the event of emergencies, but also to keep doors open for future career development. Increasingly the diversification of the roles of the HPA will offer opportunities to develop new avenues of specialist practice.

Working together

The importance of partnership between the NHS and the HPA requires ongoing efforts to enhance and improve relationships and communications. The relationship at PCT level is expressed via memoranda of understanding, which detail the links with PCT infection control staff. SHAs have responsibilities for development and monitoring all aspects of health protection, although the emergence of foundation trusts and multiple providers poses new issues to be addressed. Regional government networks extend across the range of agencies with health protection responsibilities in the wider arena than the NHS. Close working with acute hospital trusts is also important, particularly given the high burden of disease associated with hospital-acquired infections (*see* Figure 5.2).

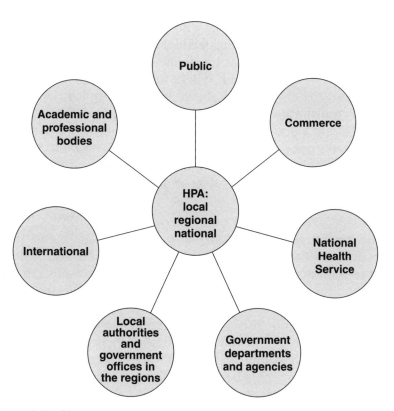

Figure 5.2: Relationships.

As part of the consultation on specialist capacity, specialists in LARS were asked to respond to a questionnaire based on issues which emerged from seminars with the minister, which were then fed into the *Choosing Health* consultation process.[8–10] Three key messages emerged.

Key messages

1 Greater clarity about roles and responsibilities

Greater clarity is needed on levels of autonomy, responsibility and accountability for health protection between PCTs, the HPA, SHAs and local government. Structural changes have created different cultures in PCTs and in the HPA. PCTs are community-based organisations with population responsibilities. The HPA has the tension of acting as a source of advice and becoming engaged in the delivery system. This is exacerbated by the lack of capacity in both PCTs and local HPA services. The horizontal/vertical tension between being part of a national system organised on hierarchical lines, and local systems with other public health colleagues makes clarity about roles and responsibilities essential. Local mapping of roles for the HPA in each locality could help to get better clarity by defining emergency planning systems with PCTs, SHAs and local government, and being clear about who should do what in response to a major incident. The potential leadership role of the SHAs needs to be developed as they are the local headquarters of the NHS. Relationships with colleagues at regional level, where links with regional government and its mechanisms reside, need also to be made explicit. Understanding the regional contribution is essential, and sharing learning opportunities can help avoid silo working and support stronger networks, particularly in areas perceived to be weak, such as ability to respond to chemical incidents. The training exercises run by the emergency response division have been found to be very useful in bridging this gap.

2 Skills and competencies

All public health staff should develop baseline skills and the competencies for health protection should be identified and reflected in training programmes. Health protection specialists are experts in different aspects of their broad portfolio, and their increasing profile and expanding remit means that the broader public health family needs a better understanding of what they do. The consultation on *Choosing Health* highlighted the need to make sure that not only all staff in the HPA but also the broader public health family including those in local government were kept up to date.[11] Developing baseline skills both in health protection and in other areas of public health would help to promote a flexible workforce across relevant organisations which was able to respond to emergencies and cover for capacity gaps. To underpin this approach, those responsible for training need to identify the competencies necessary for specialists and to develop career pathways that reflect service needs as well as professional aspirations.

3 Data

Robust data are essential to support effective practice. Improved information and availability of robust data are essential to support effective practice. For example, if the government is to be able to monitor trends in sexually transmitted diseases then systems are required to provide information to PCTs on a population basis, to enable them to trace their performance. This requires close working between health protection specialists and the NHS and observatories.

Developing specialists in health protection

HP is a rapidly developing specialty. The relevant professional bodies are in discussion about expected standards of training and their assessment. These issues of training, equivalence, standards and clinical expertise need to be considered further and clear statements made. New career pathways are emerging; for doctors *Modernising Medical Careers* offers potential for new development pathways. There are discussions about new training programmes which build on the competency-based model, allowing infectious disease, microbiology and public health sub-specialisation.[12] For other specialists the NHS *Agenda for Change* can also offer opportunities to develop new and appropriate roles to meet the health protection needs of the population.[13] Voluntary registration provides opportunities through the agreement of standards and competencies in defined areas. Further discussion will need to engage professional bodies and standard setters (*see* Chapter 3).

Gaps in skills

The *Choosing Health* consultation highlighted training and continuing professional development (CPD) needs across the breadth of public health.[10,11] Generalist specialists needed to be kept up to date with control of infection but also to learn about emergency planning, chemical and radiological hazards and other aspects of health protection. As the following quotes demonstrate, some CCDCs felt their skills were inadequate across some of these areas of health protection, and they were concerned to keep up to date with general public health:

> *There needs to be local training in place for existing consultants and specialists to keep updated in new areas such as chemical incidents, emergency planning, and radiation hazards. More joint training with environmental health officers could take place.*

Joint training for multidisciplinary working is always rewarding. There is a need for further collaboration and training with other disciplines to be more effective in these areas.

As a CCDC I would also welcome training on non-health protection general public health issues, to be kept up to speed on how to effect change for disadvantaged groups, how to get the DoH [Department of Health] to deliver a new Green Book, how to get resources from cash-strapped PCTs, etc.

Emergency planning

Emergency planning is an area of health protection practice which has received higher profile since 9/11. The capacity report highlighted the need for skills and clarity in this area with firmer national guidance on emergency planning systems relevant to all organisations, outlining clearly the respective roles of the HPA, PCTs, SHAs and regional public health groups. The Emergency Response Division of the HPA has run a series of exercises and provided advice to a wide range of people.[14]

Conclusions

Health protection is an increasingly important area of specialist practice. Threats of bioterrorism and new infectious diseases have underlined the importance of expertise in epidemiological analysis, prevention of infection and quick response to emergencies at a population level. The increasing recognition of the global nature of infections as no respecter of national boundaries, the re-emergence of infections such as TB as well as the increasing rates of sexually transmitted diseases including chlamydia, HIV/AIDS and even gonorrhoea, and the costs to healthcare of MRSA and other healthcare-acquired infections all emphasise the need for well-trained specialists with knowledge, skills and competence in health protection. The global nature of the threats and challenges also highlights why the response needs to be international.

References

1 Mandell GL, Bennett JE and Dolin R (eds) (1999) *Principles and Practices of Infectious Disease* (5e). Churchill Livingstone, Philadelphia.
2 Naylor CD, Chantler C and Griffiths S (2004) Learning from SARS in Hong Kong and Toronto. *JAMA.* **26**: 2483–7.
3 SARS Expert Committee (2003) *From Experience to Action.* SARS Expert Committee, Hong Kong.
4 Department of Health (2002) *Getting Ahead of the Curve.* Department of Health, London.

5   Health Protection Agency (2003) *Corporate Plan 2003–2008*. Health Protection Agency, London.
6   Wellcome Trust (2004) *The Challenges and Opportunities for Academic Public Health*. Wellcome Trust, London.
7   Faculty of Public Health/Health Protection Agency (2004) *On Call Guidance*. www.fph.org.uk (accessed 9 March 2005).
8   Griffiths S, Wright J and Thorpe A (2005) Public health in transition: views of the specialist workforce. Submitted to *Pub Health Med*.
9   Faculty of Public Health/Department of Health (2004) *Capacity Seminar Series – January to February 2004*. www.fph.org.uk (accessed 9 March 2005).
10 Department of Health (2004) *Choosing Health, Consultation Document*. Department of Health, London.
11 Department of Health (2004) *Choosing Health: making healthy choices easier*. Department of Health, London.
12 Department of Health (2004) *Modernising Medical Careers*. Department of Health, London.
13 Department of Health (2004) *Agenda for Change*. Department of Health, London.
14 www.hpa.org.uk (accessed 9 March 2005).

Public health in the acute setting

Chapter 6

Public health in the acute setting

Learning points

Public health specialists in hospital trusts:

- can promote joint working across primary and secondary care
- need to focus on the main business of the trust as well as on its relationships to the wider public health agenda
- need to demonstrate the economic case for their role
- can facilitate the development of basic public health skills for the wider NHS workforce, with positive benefit for staff, patients and organisational health status and outcomes
- can promote hospitals as examples of healthy workplaces.

Setting a context for public health in trusts

There are few more significant centres of activity within local communities than the hospital setting, with its patients, outpatients, visitors, professional, administrative and manual staff, and in the environment of many hospitals a growing commercial sector with shops and catering facilities serving the whole hospital community.[1]

The majority of NHS resources are committed to hospital care. Wanless challenges us to create a fully engaged scenario.[2] This includes engaging hospitals and the acute sector in public health. Events such as the severe acute respiratory syndrome (SARS) epidemic serve to highlight what can happen when the public health infrastructure is ignored (*see* Chapter 5).

The public health role of trusts is not, however, confined to control of infection, be it an acute epidemic such as SARS or a long-term challenge such as controlling hospital-acquired infections such as MRSA. Acute trusts can contribute to improving public health through:

- their contact with patients
- promoting the health of their workforce
- outreaching to their communities
- being a good corporate citizen.

In general, the public health role of NHS trusts is relatively little understood or appreciated. Very few acute trusts, and almost no mental health trusts, employ public health consultants or specialists, although those that do have been impressed by the impact made on delivery and performance. However the climate is changing, with increasing recognition that public health has a role to play across all the different sectors of healthcare.[3]

The emergence of public health in trusts

With the introduction of the internal market in 1990, most public health professionals within the NHS were employed within health authorities to provide a population perspective to health needs assessment and support the commissioning role (*see* Introduction). The first public health posts in acute hospitals were established within the Northern Region as medical care epidemiologists.[4] Regional funding was made available and trusts bid for posts. The focus of these posts was on enhancing the quality of clinical care and thereby improving outcomes.

As part of the Chief Medical Officer's (CMO's) project to strengthen the public health function in England, the Nuffield Institute for Health was commissioned to review the public health contribution to effective healthcare.[5,6] The team conducted a postal survey of all NHS trust chief executives and regional and health authority directors of public health (DPHs). This was backed up by telephone interviews with a sample of the workforce and a number of site visits. The team concluded that there was much uncertainly as to whether public health consultants should be employed in NHS trusts or whether the perceived benefits could be achieved through greater collaboration with health authorities. Greater clarification of function and roles was needed, but the need to transfer the perceived skills of public health into trusts to achieve effective healthcare was recognised.

The role and contribution of public health in trusts

There have been a number of attempts to clarify the role and functions of public health in acute trusts. In 2000 a national meeting on the role of public health and medical care epidemiologists in acute trusts spelt out key functions for the role:

- providing support to the development of clinical effectiveness guidelines and care pathways
- clinical risk management
- developing the research and development (R&D) programme and evaluating new technologies.[7]

A Department of Health-funded learning set for consultants working in acute trusts had previously identified common elements to the role and skills required.[8] These included public health specialists' engagement in spreading public health skills more widely within trusts through teaching on undergraduate and postgraduate courses for a wide range of clinicians, as well as participating in continuous professional development (CPD) arrangements for qualified staff.

A later paper produced by public health consultants working in trusts in the north in 2002 considered that to be credible within that setting, public health professionals needed to have equal standing with hospital consultants.[8] They identified the key relationship with trust medical directors. More recently, the key roles for public health specialists in trusts were described as:

- clinical governance: audit, performance management, Healthcare Commission and accreditation visits, risk management
- strategic development service planning
- trust contribution to National Service Framework (NSF) delivery, targets and demand management
- clinical effectiveness: evidence-based approaches, evaluations of services and new therapies
- R&D: mapping research output, interpretation of results, facilitating and conducting research
- leadership: bridging between clinicians and managers, change management and challenge, supporting medical director and clinical direction functions, perceived lack of bias
- health information: analysis and interpretation to shape priorities
- training and teaching: contributing to undergraduate, postgraduate and CPD programmes
- patient and public involvement: advocacy, engagement
- external role: interface with PCTs and primary care, links on commissioning.[9]

Joint work between the British Association of Medical Managers (BAMM), Faculty of Public Health and Department of Health highlighted that despite the long history, the potential role of public health specialists in hospital trusts remains largely under-developed, and under-appreciated, with those few public health specialists who do work in hospitals largely developing their own roles and contributions.

A national conference in late 2003 reviewed the role in the light of the new policy contexts as well as with particular emerging concerns about rising hospital infection rates, the potential contribution to building healthy sustainable hospitals, service redesign and modernisation and pharmaco-epidemiology.[10]

Views expressed included that public health expertise brings a scientific, epidemiological, medical and sociological perspective to acute trusts. A Chief Executive of an acute trust reported that:

> the creation of the public health post in the trust has led to critical appraisal workshops for trust board members to help them understand the evidence for clinical and policy decision making. The public health role is:
>
> - to play the honest broker in dialogue between specialties and across primary and secondary care on the development of clinical guidelines and pathways
> - to be the driving force behind many aspects of policy development particularly around clinical governance and R&D
> - to prioritise healthcare decisions by, for example, reviewing the cost-effectiveness of new drugs and new services in diabetes, stroke, lithotripsy.
>
> Our aim is that whatever we do should have a significant and beneficial impact on patient care – but it must have measurable outcomes.[11]

David Jackson

and to quote Jane Collins, Chief Executive of Great Ormond Street Hospital:

> the independent standing and ability of public health physicians to stand outside the day to day work of the acute trust and challenge the status quo is extremely important when one is trying to improve quality of services. Public health specialists focus on the needs and wants of those who use the services as opposed to the traditional way of organising things around how best to suit the professionals.[12]

A common framework for the role is being developed based on trust priorities and the wider health inequalities agenda. The competencies required have been mapped out using the Faculty of Public Health (FPH) framework, and discussions about common training in some areas of competence with medical managers have begun.

What are the ways public health can be provided in trusts?

The advantages and disadvantages of different ways of providing public health support to trusts were considered by a group of consultants from the north of England meeting in 2003. Options included:

- direct employment
- secondments from the PCT
- joint appointments.

Although all had some benefits, they concluded the greatest benefit came from direct employment because it provided greater availability and continuity and greater likelihood of working closely with hospital-based staff. Joint appointments would, however, promote collaboration across the primary and secondary care interface and engagement in new models of community-based care. Work with the BAMM and work to map delivery of public health competencies for higher specialist training within a trust setting is now being undertaken as one way to aid recruitment.[13]

What is the new agenda?

The English CMO, Sir Liam Donaldson, set a challenging agenda for public health in hospital trusts (*see* Box 6.1).

Box 6.1: Agenda for public health in hospital trusts.[9]

- To promote evidence-based clinical policy
- To promote the development of clinical governance, creating the culture, system, support and facilitation to improve quality of care, assure quality of care and improve safety
- To promote high-quality information systems, particularly trying to make these systems more population based
- The appraisal of health technology
- The reduction of infection
- The prevention of disease
- To develop pharmaco-epidemiology
- To promote the role of the NHS as a corporate citizen
- Health services research
- To re-energise the sustainability agenda, with 'green hospitals' and the 'greening' of hospitals

---

To deliver this agenda and help trusts better plan service delivery, specialists need highly developed skills in strategic thinking, political awareness, conflict resolution and communication. Key skills public health specialists can bring to the trust agenda include:

- providing a population perspective (health needs assessment, epidemiology) and supporting monitoring and audit
- interpretation of health information, using the evidence (critical appraisal, audit) to support difficult resource decisions
- health promotion and disease prevention
- clinical governance
- change management.

By focusing on the scope of the agenda, it is clear that no individual public health professional is able to do all of these things – there are not enough hours in the day. The challenge becomes how to develop a framework for public health in trusts, which can be used as a base from which to develop. As Melanie Johnson, the Minister for Public Health, said:

> Hospitals have a key role in promoting health, both as a centre of activity and also as a centre of opportunity.[1]

This is further developed in *Choosing Health*.[3]

All healthcare workers need to recognise and understand the different priorities of those who work with individuals and those who work with populations, since the optimum outcome for both groups comes from working together. Without regular face-to-face discussion, these different priorities are likely to be seen as insurmountable barriers, rather than as the source of doubly effective win–win approaches to health problems. The public health specialist can play a key role in facilitating and ensuring this dialogue takes place.

Hospitals as healthy sustainable workplaces: the challenge of the public health white paper *Choosing Health*[3]

The white paper introduces the idea of corporate social responsibility for health and calls upon the NHS to give leadership to the public sector.[3] As the country's largest employer as well as consuming local food, goods and services it can make a significant contribution to the health and sustainability of the communities served. Trusts within the NHS have, therefore, major health roles not just as employers setting examples of promoting healthy workplaces, but also as major links with local communities. In addition, commissioners have the opportunity to engage the plurality of their providers through the contract-setting process.

Views of the specialist workforce

The *Choosing Health* survey identified the need for greater emphasis to be given to the health promoting role of hospitals, including their role as employers.[14] The majority of those asked supported the proposition that monitoring of this role should be included within trust performance management arrangements. This would speed up the current slow progress and encourage greater emphasis on the public health role of hospitals:

> the NHS will have to grasp the conundrum that there is a responsibility for organisations largely commited to treating illness to address ways to prevent it

and to the lack of a formalised framework to assure delivery:

> *unless it is performance managed with the same vigour as income–expenditure balance and waiting times it is unlikely to get more than lip service . . . It is important to link this to governance arrangements (especially for foundation trusts).*

The response to the suggestion that each hospital should identify a lead person with public health clearly in their job descriptions was supported by the majority, recognition that active support of the chief executive would be a clear prerequisite of success. Seniority to exert influence across the trust was thought to be essential.

> *We need CEOs and chairs of trusts to have understanding and commitment to public health or it will remained marginalised in trusts.*

> *[It is] essential to ensure that public health cuts across all NHS services and is integral to them.*

Specialist capacity constraints mean that imaginative ways are needed to raise public health awareness in hospitals since there are not enough trained specialists for every acute trust, should they wish to employ one. Suggestions for addressing this include:

- **joint posts with PCTs**: posts shared across the primary, secondary and social care strata also reinforce the message that patients are individuals who flow through any and all parts of the NHS/social care system
- **secondments and networking arrangements**: public health capacity is limited and secondments/shared posts, or other arrangements may make best use of those skills present within an economy
- **communication of information proactively**: it is important to communicate any evidence of real benefits from trusts where this model is already used
- **long-term strategic investment in public health**: important, but invariably sidelined because of financially driven agendas
- **public health training sessions with the wider workforce**: contribution to training of others in public health skills.

Public health has a unique contribution to make to the acute trust agenda, and each health economy could begin, through combining or sharing posts, to make these skills more widely available. Placements for those in higher specialist training are a relatively untapped resource.

In summary, public health within hospitals suffered during the 1990s from the split between the providing function and the commissioning population focus of health authorities and, latterly PCTs. Those few public health specialists working in hospitals largely developed their own roles and contributions. There has been gradual clarification of the function and the part public health skills can play. It is now possible to develop a common framework for this role based on trust priorities and the wider health inequalities agenda and this has been confirmed and strengthened with the new public health white paper.[9] With the development of networks and the transfer of trust accountability to SHAs and strategic planning over whole health economies, it is easier to see how the public health role of trusts can be linked to whole-system agendas and wider health targets. However, the plurality of provision which is developing with PCT freedoms to purchase from the private sector and the establishment of foundation trusts and diagnostic and treatment centres, place new challenges for promoting public health engagement within hospitals. The possibility of shared posts, sessional commitments or secondments with wider public health input to training and CPD needs to be used to promote wider utilisation of public health skills and capacity development in the hospital sector.

References

1 Minister for Public Health (2003) Opening Speech at Public Health in Trusts Conference, October 2003, Church House, Westminster. See www.fph.org.uk

2 HM Treasury (2003) *Securing Good Health for the Whole Population*. HM Treasury, London.

3 Department of Health (2004) *Choosing Health: making healthy choices easier*. Department of Health, London.

4 Harrison S and Keen S (2002) Public health practitioners in NHS hospital trusts: the impact of medical care epidemiologists. *J Public Health*. **24**: 16–20.

5 Department of Health (2001) *The CMO's Project to Strengthen the Public Health Function*. Department of Health, London.

6 Melvin K, Wright J, Harrison SR, Robinson M and Williams DR (2000) Promoting effective practice in secondary care. *J Public Health*. **22**: 287–94.

7 The role of public health and medical care epidemiologists within trusts: report of a meeting held at the Centennial Centre, Birmingham, 24 March 2000. Unpublished.

8 The response of a group of public health practitioners in relation to the CMO's consultation process on the public health function in acute and mental health trusts. Unpublished. September 2002.

9 Faculty of Public Health (2003) *Public Health in Acute Trusts*. Report from Workshop, 3 April, Oxford Four Pillars Hotel.

10 Faculty of Public Health/British Association of Medical Managers/Department of Health (2004) *Public Health in Trusts*. Proceedings of a Workshop, May 2004, Church House, Westminster. www.fphm.org.uk/workforce/public_health_in_trusts.pdf (accessed 9 March 2005).

11 Jackson D (2004) *Public Health in Hospitals: a prerequisite for clinical excellence in public health in trusts*. Proceedings of a Workshop, May 2004, Church House, Westminster. www.fphm.org.uk/workforce/public_health_in_trusts.pdf (accessed 9 March 2005).

12 Collins J (2004) *Public Health in Trusts: all trusts need public health expertise in public health in trusts*. Proceedings of a Workshop, May 2004, Church House,

Westminster. www.fphm.org.uk/workforce/public_health_in_trusts.pdf (accessed 9 March 2005).

13   Liratsopulos G and Cook G (2003) *A Review of MFPHM Part II Competencies and RITA Portfolio Practice Areas in Relation to Public Health Training in Secondary/ Tertiary Care NHS Trusts.* March 2003. Unpublished FPH Board report.

14   Griffiths S, Wright J and Thorpe A (2005) Public health in transition: views of the specialist workforce. Submitted to *Pub Health Med.*

Tools for specialist practice

Tools for specialist practice

Learning points

This chapter describes some of the supporting 'tools' that can be used by specialists to aid practice:

- **DPH annual report**: facilitates and supports cross-sectoral working in communities
- **Health equity audits and health impact assessments**: provide specific methodologies to ensure service design and delivery and address inequalities
- Public health intelligence and surveillance systems, including public health observatories: provide evidence and inform the direction for public health programmes and delivery
- **Public health programmes**: nationally driven programmes with local implementation to bring about health gain
- **Local strategic partnerships (LSPs)**: provide a vehicle for joint work programmes on the broader health agenda
- **Using mainstream programmes/policies**
- **Delivery support**:
  - public service agreement targets
  - local delivery plans
  - monitoring performance
  - Healthcare Commission standards
- **Performance management system**: monitors and ensures delivery of key targets
- **Public health networks**: provide an infrastructure to support specialist practice.

Introduction

Previous chapters have reflected on the contribution of public health specialists in different parts of the healthcare systems and in different sectors. Perhaps uniquely among the clinical disciplines there are few, if any, areas where public health is not relevant, nor are there any sectors including local government, the voluntary sectors or business where public health approaches are not appropriate. This multidisciplinary and multisectoral nature of public health does however create its own

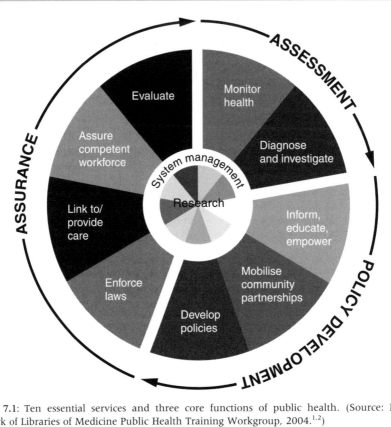

Figure 7.1: Ten essential services and three core functions of public health. (Source: National Network of Libraries of Medicine Public Health Training Workgroup, 2004.[1,2])

challenges – information needs to be collected, collated and analysed to be useful; the workforce is operating under capacity, and public health resources are scarce. The role is a busy one, as Figure 7.1 shows, and as previous chapters have emphasised.

Making sense of the agenda relies on efficient use of 'the tools' that are available to the public health specialist. Some of the key tools are described in this chapter.

The director of public health's annual report

One of the traditional areas of public health practice has been the production of an independent annual report on the state of the health of the population. Public health reports describe local data on factors that impact on health status, drawing on demographic information as well as information on broader determinants of health including housing, crime and educational attainment. The reports vary in presentational format – from data reports to videos and calendars, but all focus on addressing inequalities, influencing local government and supporting the voluntary sector as well as linking in with service delivery in the local NHS. The director of public health's (DPH's) annual report provides one mechanism for making the links between local authority and primary care trust (PCT) explicit, providing an opportunity to influence local authority members in their decision making. *Choosing Health* suggests that since the report relates to the local area, it can be used as a means of signposting areas of common interest and linking into the local strategic partnership (LSP).[3] DPHs use annual reports to audit the health status of their populations and to compare data for other geographical areas in a systematic way. The report should be presented annually to full council meetings as well as all health service partners.[4] Guidance on the content and format of these annual reports is available on the Faculty of Public Health website.[5]

Health equity audit and health impact assessment

Health equity audit (HEA) is a requirement laid out in the NHS Planning and Priorities Framework 2003–2006, and was introduced into the Healthcare Commission star ratings in 2004.[6,7] Audits are most frequently led by the Director of Public Health, providing opportunities for joined up problem solving and long-term action on complex and stubborn issues, and, in theory, supporting partnership working and the allocation of resources.[7] However, as a report by the London Health Observatory noted, they are only a requirement for the NHS, not for other sectors.[7]

A good deal of thought has been given to the process of undertaking an HEA and its uses, for example in informing local work plans, i.e. local delivery plans (LDPs) and neighbourhood renewal strategies.[8,9,10] HEAs identify how fairly resources – financial, human, and service-based – are distributed in relation to the health needs of different population groups and areas. The process can identify the priority actions required to provide services in a way that is relative to need for the population, informing the commissioning of services and contributing to local performance management of services. The aim of the audit is not to facilitate a redistribution of resources equally across the geographical patch, but rather to distribute them in a way that corresponds to the health needs of the patch, to prevent the occurrence of inequities that lead to health inequalities. As the Department of Health stresses, this is not a one-off exercise:

> *The cycle is not complete until something changes which will reduce inequalities demonstrably. For NHS services this is likely to be resource allocations, commissioning, service provision or care outcomes (p. 3).*[9]

Thus, the definition of a health equity audit relies on understanding the distinction between health inequalities and health inequity. While both terms are applied to population groups, the term 'health inequality' refers to differential experiences in health experience and health outcomes, whereas 'health inequity' describes differences in opportunity that result in unequal life chances and access to health services, etc.

More detailed information on the process and examples of their use can be found on the Association of Public Health Observatories website.[11]

Health impact assessment (HIA) is a new tool to assess the impact on health of policies affecting the public. It can apply to any new development or change of policy or service where there is a potential positive or negative effect on the health of the public. HIA aims to ensure health inequalities are either reduced, or at least not widened by policy or service change, providing a structured process to review evidence, gather information, consult with all stakeholders including affected members of the public, and inform the decision-making process. There are a number of different methodologies and HIA toolkits to support specialists ranging from detailed research protocols to HIA by rapid appraisal.[12] The HIA Gateway suggests that they are characterised by a six-stage process, as detailed in Box 7.1.

Box 7.1: Six steps to an HIA (adapted from the HIA Gateway[13])

1 **Screening**: deciding which proposals require assessment by HIA
2 **Scoping**: defining the parameters
3 **Appraisal and assessment**: identifying and analysing the potential impact of the proposal on health
4 **Developing** recommendations to improve the proposal, including addressing the issue of inequalities
5 **Active engagement** in adapting proposals
6 **Monitoring and evaluating** the impact of the adaptations and their implementation

---

For further information on the concepts, processes and uses of HIAs the Health Impact Assessment Gateway is an invaluable resource. Examples of HIAs which have been undertaken can be accessed on the website.[12]

Local strategic partnerships

The LSPs, and their associated partnerships, are a vehicle which can help set a common agenda to improve health and reduce inequalities through the health services and local government for a given population. As *The NHS Improvement Plan* said:

> *These partnerships facilitate greater co-ordination in delivering health and social care services to local populations. . . . (p. 51).*[14]

Members of the LSP come from many organisations apart from PCTs and local councils, each bringing specific expertise and abilities to the LSP to address common agendas. Developing these structures may encourage the development of closer cross-institutional links, and thus impact positively on public health, providing the partnerships are given the appropriate time and support to 'settle' and develop relationships (*see* Box 7.2). *Raising Health* suggests that LSPs provide a vehicle for integrating work across the organisational boundaries by facilitating a focus on population groupings and on settings, i.e. schools, nurseries, etc.[15] This focus can provide a filter for identifying partners and effective interventions, with a potential for pooled budgets, information and other resources to achieve a common aim. However, as *Raising Health* suggested, the differing performance management frameworks and targets that the members of the LSPs were subjected to influence the areas of work which are given priority by the members of the group.[1]

Box 7.2: Tips from local strategic partnerships for flexible use of resources across sectors (source: Health Development Agency, 2004)[16]

- Clarify the common objectives and rationale for pooling resources.
- Explore partners' perceptions of the process and expected outcomes.
- Agree who contributes, the type of resources to be combined, how much, for how long, and with what management and accountability arrangements.
- Draw up accountability agreements/protocols setting out the roles and responsibilities of the partners involved, and how risk will be managed if there are problems.
- Focus on specific community strategy priorities, themes or geographic areas where the LSP can add value by co-ordinating its resources to achieve local targets.
- It can be easier to pilot pooled arrangements by combining externally acquired funds initially, before pooling mainstream resources, staff or services.
- If specific grants are pooled, check that the conditions of use can be satisfied by the lead agency for the grant.
- Cross-sector information and communication across financial systems are essential for effective management of pooled resources across the LSP.
- Finance directors, elected members and agency lawyers will be key players in championing new approaches and in advocating the use of pooled resources to chief executives and service managers – their knowledge of existing flexibilities and a positive approach to experimentation will be critical.
- The lessons and outcomes of pooling resources can be shared between LSP partnerships to support a common approach.

One of the key challenges is to ensure that the agendas are common to all partners. The Department of Health has a responsibility to input into this process – as it acknowledges:

> . . . the Department of Health will work to align strategies, priorities, objectives and targets more closely across other government departments, including shared objectives to maximise consistency and ensure effective delivery (Chapter 4).[14]

This theme runs through the approach to delivering the agenda set in *Choosing Health*, which stresses the need to align investment, performance assurance mechanisms, planning guidance, inspection and regulation between local government and the NHS.[3] Steps are being taken to achieve this not only through the already published public service agreement (PSA) targets,[17] but also the technical LDP guidance. In addition, local government will be able to use the new requirement for local PSAs (LPSAs) and build on the experience of local area agreements (LAAs) where merged funding has been piloted

Public health intelligence and surveillance systems

Specialist skills in health intelligence are an essential component of public health practice, enabling systematic analysis of data from a range of sources. However, as Wanless noted:

> there is no regular mechanism by which a PCT or local authority can gather reliable information on its own population (p. 107).[1]

This issue was addressed in *Choosing Health*, which suggested that although building blocks were in place:

> they do not yet add up to a coherent information system geared to today's needs (p. 191).[3]

To rectify this situation, the report announced the establishment of a Health Information and Intelligence Task Force with nine key tasks (*see* Box 7.3).

Box 7.3: Tasks of Health Information and Intelligence Taskforce (adapted from Annex B, *Choosing Health*, p. 191)[3]

1 Develop real-time public health information leading to action at a local level.
2 Identify an agreed set of core data to support agreed measures of progess.
3 Tackle weaknesses within existing data.

4 Bring together sources of information on health and wellbeing from routine sources and local studies, to give a comprehensive picture of how lifestyle factors affect health (*see* Box 7.4).

5 Work with the Health Protection Agency (HPA) to develop effective systems.

6 Use new sources, such as marketing information and systems of information to improve the health of the population.

7 Give guidance on data sharing and on disclosure and confidentiality.

8 Build on existing knowledge management systems to promote best practice.

9 Build on the work of the public health observatories on regional public health indicators to establish a framework for health surveillance at a regional level, which supports a more robust national framework.

Box 7.4: Sources of routine information

- Public health observatories
- Registers
- Health Protection Agency (HPA)
- National Programme for Information Technology

The role of public health observatories

Originally established following *Saving Lives*, public health observatories operate at a regional level, their remit being to provide information on health in its broadest sense and draw together data from a very wide range of sources.[18] *Choosing Health* emphasises the importance of their role in contributing to partnerships and networks.[3] Their role is being expanded to provide more support for PCTs not only in their commissioning roles but also in analysis of local data. For further information see the Association of Public Health Observatories website.[19]

Cancer registries also span large population bases and have been collecting and providing data on new registrations and trends in mortality from different cancers since the 1980s. These data have proved invaluable in targeting service effort. For further information on their role, see the Association of Cancer Registries website.[20]

The HPA runs a number of different surveillance systems on communicable disease data, ranging from sexual health to monitoring infectious disease outbreaks. The National Communicable Disease Surveillance

Centre is crucial in bringing together information from local services, health protection teams and laboratories around the country. For example, the HPA's recent information on trends in sexual health diseases highlighting increasing rates of HIV/AIDS and chlamydia has been instrumental in influencing the government's policy and establishment of new targets for services as part of the *Choosing Health* white paper.[3] While the role of the HPA was not explicitly mentioned in the white paper, the delivery plan needs to reflect the contribution of all elements of the public health workforce, i.e. health protection and academic roles as well as health improvement, health protection and health service support/ research, to ensure a comprehensive and mainstream approach to health improvement. (For further information on the role of the HPA, *see* Chapter 5 and the HPA website.[21])

Other opportunities for improving access to information and the evidence base are offered by the new National Programme for Information Technology for the NHS. As the *Better Information, Better Choices, Better Health* white paper suggests, the role of this programme in collaboration with other initiatives, in improving access by signposting quality information, is considerable – both for the public and for the NHS professional.[22] It enables faster learning and ensures that proven models can be put into practice more rapidly than ever before.

Using mainstream programmes/policies, e.g. chronic disease management and the GP contract

Throughout this book, we have emphasised the multidisciplinary nature of public health. The changes in contractual arrangements for doctors, pharmacists, etc provide a further vehicle to drive forward the public health agenda.

Box 7.5: Care provision: an overview (adapted from Annex B, *Choosing Health*, p. 205)[3]

Nationally agreed general medical services (GMS) contract used by 60% of general practice:

- obliges practices to provide essential services for those who are ill or believe themselves to be ill, and chronic disease management and appropriate health promotion
- additional services provided by the majority of practices, e.g. flu jabs
- enhanced services provided by many practices, e.g. drug abuse services, often by a practitioner with a special interest.

Personal medical services (PMS): a more locally sensitive model, with contract agreed with the PCT. May provide quite specialised services in primary care settings, e.g. for the homeless.

Direct PCT provision where locally necessary e.g. direct employment of a general practitioner (GP) to support care of people with many health problems.

Alternative provider medical services whereby a PCT can contract for provision of any necessary care for its population with the private, voluntary, or charitable sectors, alone or in partnership with each other or other NHS providers.

All contracting routes will offer well-organised care that can be monitored through the **Quality and Outcomes Framework (QOF)**.

The proposed **new pharmacy contract** will reflect the public health role of pharmacists both within the essential services component of the contract and the locally commissioned enhanced services.

The changes in care provision offer considerable scope for developing mainstream commitment to the public health agenda (*see* Box 7.5).

Public health programmes and their delivery

The Labour government of the late 1990s introduced the concept of National Service Frameworks (NSFs) as the vehicle for driving national health policy for different disease areas and reducing geographical inequity in delivery and quality of care. To date, NSFs have been issued covering cancer, coronary heart disease, mental health, older people, diabetes and children's services. More are pending. Each spans prevention to tertiary care with standards and targets, based on best evidence, for each activity.

The *NHS Improvement Plan* built on this approach by setting out a comprehensive agenda for a modernised NHS (*see* Figure 7.2).[14]

The plan calls for a radical reconceptualisation of the NHS, prioritising preventative public health measures:

> the NHS will be able to concentrate on transforming itself from a sickness service to a health service. Prevention of disease and tackling inequalities in health will assume a much greater priority in the NHS. With the NHS working in partnership with others and with individuals to support people in choosing healthier approaches to their lives, real progress will be made on preventing ill health and reducing inequalities in health (p. 14).[14]

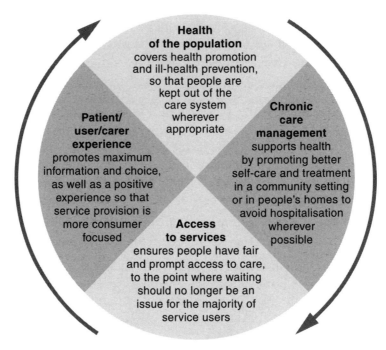

Figure 7.2: Future objectives for the NHS. (Source: Department of Health, 2004.[14])

This has been further re-emphasised by *Choosing Health* which stresses the shift of emphasis within the NHS from health services to health – at the same time as reinforcing the opportunities for the acute hospital system to promote health as described earlier in Chapter 6.[3] The important thing to note here is the shift in emphasis.

The National Service Frameworks for both cancer and heart disease are committed to reducing the harm created by smoking tobacco, diets low in fruit and vegetables, lack of physical activity and abuse of alcohol. However, as *Choosing Health* states:

> *existing health improvement and prevention approaches need to be adapted to maximise their impact and to mainstream a comprehensive approach to health improvement across the NHS from primary care, through hospital care to specialist services and all clinical settings (p. 122).*[3]

The challenge spelt out advocates achieving this greater focus on prevention through:

- partnership working across all the sectors
- communications building on previous successful campaigns
- raising awareness of health risks with information about action that people can take themselves to address those risks
- engaging all NHS staff in this endeavour.

Box 7.6: Programme commitments in *Choosing Health*[3]

- **Sexual health:** a new national campaign targeted particularly at younger men and women to ensure that they understand the real risk of unprotected sex, and persuade them of the benefits of using condoms to avoid the risk of sexually transmitted infections (STIs) or unplanned pregnancies.
- **Obesity:** a new cross-government campaign to raise awareness of the health risks of obesity, and the steps people can take through diet and physical activity to prevent obesity.
- **Smoking:** a boosted campaign to reduce smoking rates and motivate smokers in different groups to quit, supported by clear and comprehensive information about health risks, reasons not to smoke, and access to NHS support to quit, including 'stop smoking' services and nicotine replacement therapy.
- **Alcohol:** working with the Portman Group* to cut down binge drinking.

Specialist public health expertise can and does assist in providing evidence of effective interventions, organising and supporting programmes – e.g. the existing smoking cessation programme – evaluating their impact (*see* Box 7.6).

Performance management: LDP lines/PSA targets

National policy and the drive to change practice need to be underpinned by performance management systems relating to key targets. This ensures a consistency in approach across the country and also that all organisations are addressing the same priorities. Throughout this book we have referred to some of the mechanisms by which performance management takes place, for example public sector agreements shared between health and local government, and the balanced scorecard approach by which standards in PCTs and hospital trusts are measured. Public health is one of the seven domains of core and developmental outcomes set out in the new Planning Framework *National Standards, Local Action* published in July 2004:[23]

> *Programmes and services are designed and delivered in collaboration with all relevant organisations and communities to promote, protect and improve the health of the population serviced and reduce health inequalities between different population groups and areas.*

---

*The Portman Group (www.portman-group.org.uk) is an organisation set up in 1989 by the UK's leading drinks producers to promote responsible drinking, marketing and a balanced understanding of alcohol-related issues.

Box 7.7: Features of the system (source: Department of Health, 2005[24])

- A shift to a system where standards of quality and care across the full spectrum of healthcare and all age groups act as the key national driver for improvements.
- Progress against standards will be independently assessed by the Healthcare Commission and will inform performance ratings from April 2005.
- A reduced set of national targets to accelerate progress in a small number of priority areas, with particular focus on improving the health of the population.
- Characterised by increasing focus on health outcomes rather than service input.
- More headroom for local prioritisation.
- Financial and performance assessment incentives aligned to support improvement in the system.
- Local organisations taking a greater lead in service modernisation.

Local delivery plans

The most recent guidance on performance management relating to the next planning and assessment round introduces more flexibility to allow for locally sensitive targets to meet local health needs (*see* Boxes 7.7 and 7.8).

Box 7.8: Organisation responsibilities

Primary care trusts:

- commission services and set LDPs
- account to SHAs through LDPs for achieving levels of performance.

Strategic health authorities:

- agree and sign off levels of performance set in LDPs
- provide support to manage improvements.

Department of Health:

- signs off SHA-level plans, ensuring that national performance expectations are formally agreed and disaggregated to both SHA and PCT levels
- provides support to SHAs who are under-performing against the plan – instigating recovery and support arrangements only where there is significant under-performance by the SHA.

The LDP is a key reference point for the Healthcare Commission to use in determining 'star ratings'.

Local targets

One of the main aims of the reduction in new national targets is to create greater headroom for organisations to set locally appropriate targets. While there are no mandatory requirements for target setting, there are six key principles (*see* Box 7.9).

Box 7.9: Principles for local target setting[23]

Targets should:

- be in line with population needs
- address local service gaps
- deliver equity
- be evidence based
- be developed in partnership with other NHS organisations and local authorities
- offer value for money.

The delivery plan for *Choosing Health* is one of the national resources which PCTs and local authorities can draw upon in setting their local targets and LAAs.[3] LAAs provide models for more flexible and responsive arrangements and relationships between central government and local communities. In total, there are 21 pilot LAAs, which will draw their priorities from the PSAs on children and young people, safer and stronger communities, and healthier communities and older people.[24] For more information on LAAs, see the Local Government Vision website.[25]

Supporting public health specialists: the role of public health networks

The concept of the managed public health network entered the public policy arena with *Shifting the Balance of Power: securing delivery* (p. 46).[26] This document formalised the need for PCTs to assume responsibility for assessing the health needs of their local communities – linking delivery explicitly with notions of partnership, i.e.

> by PCTs co-operating through public health networks to pool resources and talent (p. 13).[26]

The purpose of the network was therefore to make better use of skills that were being dispersed through the restructuring process, and to facilitate the pooling of resources to cover areas that were best dealt with at a supra-PCT level. The *Capacity Seminars* and *Choosing Health* surveys demonstrated considerable variation in the structure of public health networks, on a spectrum from the highly organised and well co-ordinated managed network to informal information sharing without any specific infrastructural support.[4,27] However, as Fahey (2003) notes, these differences are hidden behind a tendency to talk about 'networks' as though they are a single entity.[28]

Networks nationally are characterised by diversity of:

- managerial forms
- the formality of the business plans and workload
- staffing
- levels of commitment from the locality in which they are based
- availability of staffing
- financial standings.

This diversity of forms is matched by a diversity of opinion about the need to clarify the roles and functions for networks.[29]

Many PCTs have experienced difficulties in recruiting to DPH posts; mobility of the workforce is still high, and single-handed practice is not uncommon. However, the conundrum remains that the PCTs that have larger teams have the capacity to be self-sufficient and therefore do not need to network to deliver their local objectives, whereas small teams and single-handed DPHs need network help to deliver on the public health agenda, but cannot contribute the time and resource to the development of the network.

This is difficult where resources are not equitably distributed across PCTs. The DPH must put their own PCT first and must sustain credibility with their chief executive. The network has to come second to this.[4]

For PCTs to engage with this, there is an obvious need to demonstrate benefits from membership of the network in terms of delivery of key objectives, and substantive benefit to the PCT.

> *Hard to prioritise network work over PCT work if you can't demonstrate the local value of this.*[4]

> *There are so many opportunities within PCTs that I am reluctant to pull people out for network activities unless it is really essential – it is better to keep a strong PCT base.*[4]

With the continuing move towards a primary care locus of control for health service commissioning, managed public health networks have the potential to facilitate the sharing of common approaches between PCTs for issues which are best addressed across larger populations, thus avoiding duplication of work and fragmentation of resources, for example in the commissioning of specialist services.

The need for partnership working, via public health networks, in order to deliver the public health agenda has been explicitly mandated in numerous policy documents.[18] While networks, where they are functioning well, have increased public health capacity and capabilities by providing frameworks for delivery and professional support, 58.5% of respondents to the *Choosing Health* survey supported a need for explicit central guidance if the full value of the network approach is to be achieved.[4]

The issue of communication to promote network functionality is addressed by Jessop.[30] He suggests that routine reports, regular meetings and rapid response to queries are essential components of the successful network. While electronic networks facilitate the effective functioning of the network, they do not act as a replacement for face-to-face meetings. His suggestion was for the network to hold one meeting per month, with regular attendance being required of all network members. However, the practicalities of this in a climate of deadlines, increasing workloads and a fragmented and geographically diverse organisation are open to question. There is however a need to ensure effective communication, and to ensure a coherent work plan for the network if it is to achieve legitimacy and buy-in from its stakeholder organisations.

Choosing Health further reinforces the need to develop managed public health networks as key mechanisms to support partnership work and organisations by providing highly specialised and essential public health skills, and PCTs are charged, in partnership with their local organisations and local authorities, to proactively manage specialist public health services and functions across the whole community.[3] Lessons should be learned from clinical networks where investing in an infrastructure, management information research and governance as well as clinical leadership has led to a step change in delivery (para 79 annex b).

Conclusion

As this book has affirmed throughout, meeting the new health challenges of the 21st century will require a step change in action. With the positive policy climate, the new tools and the new regulatory frameworks, the position of public health is increasingly being recognised as mainstream. The role of the public health specialist is to take best advantage of this, to demonstrate that sustained and focused action can and does improve people's health. The opportunity is there – it is up to public health to take it, before it disappears.

References

1 HM Treasury (2004) *Securing Health for the Whole Population*. HM Treasury, London.

2 National Network of Libraries of Medicine Public Health Training Workgroup (2004) *Public Health Information and Data: a training manual*. http://phpartners.org/pdf/phmanual.pdf (accessed 11 March 2005).

3 Department of Health (2004) *Choosing Health: making healthy choices easier*. Department of Health, London.

4 Griffiths S, Wright J and Thorpe A (2005) Public health in transition: views of the specialist workforce. Submitted to *Pub Health Med*.

5 www.fph.org.uk (accessed 11 March 2005).

6 Department of Health (2002) *Improvement, Expansion and Reform: the next three years' priorities and planning framework 2003–2006*. Department of Health, London.

7 Aspinall P and Jacobson B (2005) Pre-publication draft. *Health Equity Audit: a baseline survey of PCTs*. www.lho.org.uk/Health_Inequalities/Attachments/Word_Files/Health_Equity_Audit_Final_Report.doc (accessed 11 March 2005).

8 Hamer L, Jacobson B, Flowers J and Johnson F (2003) *Health Equity Audit Made Simple: a briefing for primary care trusts and local strategic partnerships*. HDA, London.

9 Department of Health (2005) *Health Equity Audit: a guide for the NHS*. www.dh.gov.uk/assetRoot/04/08/41/39/04084139.pdf (accessed 11 March 2005).

10 Whitehead M (1992) The concepts and principles of equity in health. *Int J Health Serv*. **22**(3): 429–45.

11 www.apho.org.uk (accessed 11 March 2005).

12 The HIA Gateway www.hiagateway.org.uk (accessed 11 March 2005).

13 www.hiagateway.org.uk/beginners/beginner_three.htm (accessed 11 March 2005).

14 Department of Health (2004) *The NHS Improvement Plan: putting people at the heart of public services*. Department of Health, London. www.dh.gov.uk/assetRoot/04/08/45/22/04084522.pdf (accessed 11 March 2005).

15 Office of Public Management (2004) *Raising Health*. Office of Public Management, London.

16 Health Development Agency (2004) *Pooling Resources Across Sectors*. www.lga.gov.uk/download.asp?path=/Documents/Briefing/Our_Work/BLG/pooling.pdf (accessed 11 March 2005).

17 HMT (2004) *2004 Spending Review*. HMT, London. www.hm-treasury.gov.uk

18 Department of Health (1999) *Saving Lives: our healthier nation*. Department of Health, London.

19 www.apho.org.uk (accessed 11 March 2005).

20 www.ukacr.org.uk (accessed 11 March 2005).

21 www.hpa.org.uk (accessed 11 March 2005).

22 Department of Health (2004) *Better Information, Better Choices, Better Health: putting information at the heart of health*. Department of Health, London.

23 Department of Health (2004) *National Standards, Local Action*. Department of Health, London.

24 Department of Health (2005) *Choosing Health: management, inspection and assessment of performance*. Department of Health, London.

25 www.odpm.gov.uk/localvision (accessed 11 March 2005).

26 Department of Health (2001) *Shifting the Balance of Power: securing delivery*. Department of Health, London.

27 Faculty of Public Health/Department of Health/PHRU (2004) *Capacity Seminars*. January and February 2004. FPH, London.

28 Fahey D (2003) *The Public Health Network: a systemic and model-based approach*. MSc in Health Informatics Dissertation, City University, London.

39 Pedler M (2001) *Issues in Health Development. Networked organisations: an overview*. NHS Confederation, London.

30 Jessop E (2002) Leading and managing public health networks. *J Public Health Med*. **24**(3): 240.

Looking to the future

Chapter 8

Looking to the future

So far in the preceding chapters we have described the current roles and perspectives on specialist public health practice. Specialist practice is now fully multidisciplinary and is developing rapidly. The policy context for specialist practice in England remains positive, reinforced by the white paper, action to reduce second-hand smoke and a growing awareness of the importance of infectious disease as well as the burden of chronic disease related to obesity. All this poses challenges for training, careers and responsibilities for leadership at all levels of the system.

But what of the future?

Professional structures

The basis of professional education within public health is now based on an approach common to other professions. For those considering a career as a specialist there is now a deeper, if still developing, understanding of:

- a common multidisciplinary framework for basic generalist training, based on modern educational principles
- clear entry criteria for acceptance into training
- a structured training framework which is modular and flexible
- defined areas of competence assessed through demonstration of knowledge, skills, attitudes and expertise in areas spelt out in curriculae
- ongoing appraisal of practice to ensure standards are maintained
- registration to protect the public
- ongoing professional development with a commitment to lifelong learning, including the development of the 'skills escalator' for public health.

These pieces of the professional jigsaw are still being shaped, and the overall picture will continue to change, influenced by external forces such as service requirements and policy initiatives, as well as professional influences including the implementation of policies from the Postgraduate Medical and Education Training Board (PMETB) and the *Agenda for Change* initiatives, themselves responding to the modernisation of healthcare practice.[1]

New careers

The future shape of specialist practice will be influenced by national initiatives which include those influencing other parts of the NHS work-force. They include:

Modernising Medical Careers and the PMETB

The structural changes within postgraduate medical education are relevant to public health, signalled within policies such as *Modernising Medical Careers* which proposes changes to the early career pathways for doctors.[2] *Modernising Medical Careers* introduces foundation years with rotations which will give experience of a menu of options within medicine.[2] Public health will be included within some of these. Doctors hoping to specialise in public health will then be able to join specialist training programmes that will provide the opportunity for cumulative acquisition and assessment of competence within the curriculum as agreed with the PMETB. Ongoing attachments and rotational posts within specialist train-ing will also allow a combination of public health experience and experi-ence of other specialties such as paediatrics, general practice and health protection. In future it may well be that new career pathways to specialist practice will emerge, which include clinical and public health components in new combinations. One example that is under discussion is the creation of health protection specialist careers which combine experience/practice of microbiology, infectious disease and public health. These medical career pathways will be recognised under the auspices of the PMETB.[3]

The PMETB has replaced the Specialist Training Authority as the body which can certificate doctors at the end of their training. It is responsible for standards, curriculae and training for doctors, working closely with the royal colleges and the NHS to train doctors to both UK and European standards.

Flexible training

Another element of modern thinking which offers opportunities for new ways of practice is the commitment within both medicine and all other healthcare professions to flexible training which can be lifelong and incremental. This is often expressed as a 'skills escalator'.

Our approach to workforce development therefore needs to reflect the philosophy of lifelong learning and flexible careers based on acquisition of competencies. Extending the approach to encourage the acquisition of competencies in defined areas will also give formal recognition of the contribution that key professionals, e.g. pharmacists, psychologists, public health information analysts, academics, health promotion professionals etc, can make at practitioner and specialist levels. This will not only broaden considerably the base of specialist practice but also bring in professionals based in organisations beyond the health service. This has implications for funding of training and how that is managed across sectors, as well as introducing the need to widen the base of specialist trainers.

Skills escalator

The 'skills escalator' or 'climbing frame' is a model for education which incorporates development of modular assessment and accreditation against explicit standards. It is one which, following the white paper, needs further development (*see* Figure 8.1).[4]

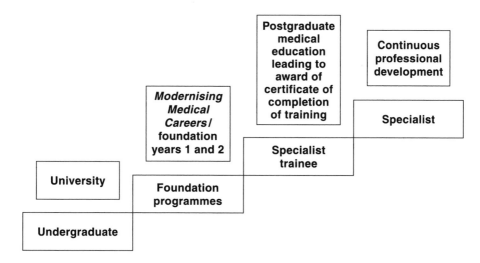

Figure 8.1: Example of the 'skills escalator': medical career pathway.

Career pathways need to be developed at all levels of practice within the NHS and beyond, in discussion with professional groups, educators, registering bodies, employers and the public. This approach should underpin any approach to developing the public health workforce, and is one to which the NHS University (NHSU) or its replacement body, the National Institute for Learning Skills and Innovation (NILSI), is uniquely suited, given its national remit – albeit that its specific role is yet to be clarified at the time of writing.

As part of this approach, the contribution of defined competencies to the development of a career framework for public health has been explored in two workshops hosted by the NHSU in November 2004 and January 2005 respectively. Competencies have been developed at both practitioner and specialist levels for public health by Skills for Health.[5] They provide a broad definition of good practice, and a framework which is transferable and transparent – but not large amounts of detail, which enables flexibility in their use across professional groupings. The benefits of this approach were felt to be the promotion of a coherent overview of the public health workforce, facilitation of a multisectoral approach, and use of a shared language which enabled transfer to contexts, e.g. to environmental health officers, and to other contexts of work. The standards were formally approved in February 2004, and published in March 2004. They can be accessed on the Skills for Health website.[6]

However, standards are not the whole answer, but rather need to be considered in conjunction with other aspects – for example in the context of a career framework. The example of the Scottish Partnership work illustrates the ways in which taking a competency approach had been utilised in Scotland to develop a functional map for public health, which could be used as a tool for organisational planning.[7]

The career escalator approach fits well with the *Knowledge and Skills Framework* (KSF),[8] advocated by *Agenda for Change*,[1] which focuses on the ability to use knowledge and skills in a role, relating this to pay progression. The KSF is not about competencies *per se*, although it is explicit that they link in, and is the end result of a large partnership process, including unions. It has been nationally agreed with the four UK countries for the NHS.

The white paper commitment to 'develop training and support for all NHS staff to develop their understanding and skills in promoting health' provides an impetus for a comprehensive and co-ordinated work programme to design a national public health curriculum to deliver these objectives. The Changing Workforce programme's *Career Framework* document aims to provide a guide for NHS and partner organisations on the implementation of a flexible career and skills escalator concept, enabling an individual with transferable, competency-based skills to progress in a direction which meets workforce, service and individual needs – across nine levels of the public health workforce.[9] Details of the programme can be found on the NHS Modernisation Agency website.[10]

Registering equivalence

At a time when registration of professionals is being reviewed as part of the government's arm's-length bodies review, the future of public health registration is also under consideration.[11] As one of the actions in *Our Healthier Nation*, the Voluntary Register for public health specialists was established in May 2003.[12,13] It aims to publish a list of competent specialists in public health, and thorough periodic revalidation to ensure specialists in public health keep up to date and maintain competence, and deal with registered specialists who fail to meet the necessary standards.

Discussions have been taking place with all registering bodies about how specialist standards can be developed on the basis of equivalence between registers, to reflect shared standards of practice and their assurance under the auspices of the evolving Council for Healthcare Regulatory Excellence (CHRE).[14]

One model that has been proposed is for each registering body to identify the equivalent level of competence for specialists within their professional group, not only at specialist level but also at practitioner level. For example, both the General Medical Council (GMC) and the General Dental Council (GDC) have recognised the professional standards proposed by the Faculty of Public Health (FPH). Formally these were also the standards agreed with the Specialist Training Authority but will in future need to be signed off by the PMETB. There is also potentially a new role for the CHRE to take an overview of the registration for public health on existing registers such as the Nursing and Midwifery Council (NMC), GMC and GDC. All those not on existing professional registers would be able to register via the Voluntary Register, which could in time become statutory, and which ensures equivalence of standards expected by other registering bodies.

Developing the concept of public health leadership

Our theme throughout the book has been of the public health specialist as an independent professional able to operate and lead within and across a wide range of organisations. The *Choosing Health* consultation identified that the biggest gap in meeting challenging new public health agendas was the need for leadership training.[15] Specialists, particularly directors of public health (DPHs), need to no longer sit on the sidelines offering advice, but to get engaged with their communities and provide leadership for health. Academics need to re-engage with service colleagues and provide evidence of effective interventions.

Roemer has described the requirements for public health leadership as:

- knowledge of public health problems and the content of public health action programmes
- basic education and experience
- organisational and administrative support (guidance, consultation, etc) in a hierarchical structure
- training in management
- practical experience in management
- adequate physical resources
- a favourable moral or spiritual environment.[16]

The Medical Leadership development programme for medical directors in the programme for the NHS Leadership Centre has suggested that the key areas for development are:

- understanding the challenges of the role
- understanding the national policy agenda: the imperatives and drivers of change in a modern NHS
- understanding governance
- developing local networks
- finding creative approaches to problem solving – including how to reframe decisions and problems
- aligning personal and organisational goals.[17]

The workshops run by the Leadership Centre and the FPH agreed that the leadership roles of DPHs need to include:

- communication
- teamworking/partnership working
- handling the tension between advocacy and the corporate role
- managing upwards
- playing a role in the delivery culture
- focusing on performance management
- developing personal networks, identifying the power brokers to influence and delivering at each level.[18]

Suggestions for delivery mechanisms put forward by the *Choosing Health* consultation process included:

- mentoring: by a public health person, by a management mentor, by an experienced chief executive officer (CEO), peer group, consumer-based mentoring, i.e. by general practitioners (GPs) – while reflections on this were largely positive, one respondent suggested that 'mentoring is sticking plaster for a wound that will not heal without radical surgery'
- coaching
- leadership courses for directors
- DPH learning sets
- job experience: a 'followership role' for corporate duties
- buddying for new starters
- formal continuing professional development (CPD) programmes, not limited to DPHs
- personal development plans.[19]

These skills need to play into specialist public health practice wherever it takes place. Leadership skills need to form a key part of higher specialist training and practitioner development.[3]

If we are to see a step change in effectiveness of specialists in public health we ignore these needs at our peril.

International working

While this book has concentrated on public health specialist practice in England, there is a growing awareness of the need to work not only within Europe to develop common approaches to training and professional practice, but also wider afield. European legislation has a direct impact on the training of doctors working and training in public health, because of the legislative requirements of the European Union (EU). The law assumes for all public health doctors that they are able to apply to work in all parts of the EU without further qualification, as long as they can demonstrate achievement of equivalent standards of experience and competence as judged through their national systems. This area of work needs to be better understood, particularly in the light of the expanding membership of the EU.

There are other agreements for some other professional groups, e.g. nurses who come from the EU/EEA have a right to practise in the UK,[20] but the unique situation of multidisciplinary public health means both legislative and logistical difficulties in translating the UK system to other countries.

The role of the royal colleges and hence of the faculty of public health is particular to the UK. It is more closely emulated in some of the (old) commonwealth countries but others including the US tend to accredit qualifications and their awarding bodies, such as Schools of Public Health, not individual training programmes. Thus the qualification of a Masters in Public Health in the US is in itself a qualification, whereas in the UK it is the certification to practise, based on having shown a level of competence that counts to designate specialist status. However, there is much to learn from the competency-based models which are increasingly being used to support the development of the public health workforce.[21]

For example, the US Association of Schools of Public Health supports a Public Health Centers-networked training programme to strengthen the technical, scientific, managerial and leadership competence of the current and future public health workforce.[22] It has five key activities:

1 developing an academic and practice collaborative to promote workforce development
2 assessing training needs
3 developing training resources
4 providing training programmes
5 evaluating the impact of training.

The core competencies of individuals it aims to promote are in seven skills areas:

1 analysis/assessment/policy development/programme planning
2 communication
3 cultural competency
4 community dimensions of practice
5 public health sciences
6 financial planning
7 management leadership and systems thinking.

These domains underpin the work led by Gebbie in producing the competency to curriculum toolkit supported by the Association of Teachers of Preventive Medicine.[21]

The experience of severe acute respiratory syndrome (SARS) highlighted the global nature of disease and it also demonstrated the lack of investment in the public health infrastructure.[23] An effectively trained public health workforce with the necessary expertise and skills is essential not only for combating acute epidemics but also dealing with the chronic problems associated with obesity, heart disease, poverty and pollution. Just as public health issues are common across national boundaries, so too are the learning needs of the workforce. To quote the Institute of Medicine (IOM) report in the US:

> regardless of their backgrounds, public health professionals must have a framework for action and an understanding of the forces that impact on health, a model of health that emphasizes the linkages and relationships among multiple determinants affecting health.[24]

Future collaboration across international boundaries must be the way to go.

Conclusion

Inevitably, since the FPH sets specialist public health standards, we have dwelt on the work we are aware of over the past years as the profession has moved from its medical to its multidisciplinary base. We have highlighted the opportunities created by the changes, the direction of travel and some of the issues that need to be addressed if we are to see a thriving profession. The complexities of working between professions within the NHS are not to be underestimated as we move toward a stronger multidisciplinary base. There are the additional complexities of working with other sectors particularly those in local government and within academe, continually redefining the skills and competencies required for new ways of working. The rapidly expanding remit of health protection demonstrates the need to continually push the boundaries of specialist practice. We have drawn from the views of the specialists who responded to the *Choosing Health* consultation and from UK-wide events in recent years,[19] and in doing so have provided a benchmark for measuring both the progress made and the milestones we need to reach.

References

1 Department of Health (2001) *Agenda for Change*. Department of Health, London.
2 Department of Health (2004) *Modernising Medical Careers: the next steps*. Department of Health, London.
3 www.pmetb.org.uk/pmetb (accessed 11 March 2005).
4 Department of Health (2004) *Choosing Health: making healthy choices easier*. Department of Health, London.
5 Skills for Health (2004) *National Occupational Standards for the Practice of Public Health: Guide, March 2004*. Skills for Health, Bristol.
6 www.skillsforhealth.org.uk (accessed 11 March 2005).
7 Scottish Partnership Project (2004) *Joint Report: occupational standards/ competences for public health practice*. Health Scotland, Edinburgh. www.healthscotland.com (accessed 11 March 2005).
8 Department of Health (2004) *Knowledge and Skills Framework*. Department of Health, London.
9 Modernisation Agency (2004) *Career Framework for the NHS*. www.modern.nhs.uk/scripts/default.asp?site_id=65&id=24529 (accessed 11 March 2005).
10 www.modern.nhs.uk (accessed 11 March 2005).
11 Department of Health (2004) *Reconfiguring the Department of Health's Arm's Length Bodies: implementation framework*. Department of Health, London.
12 Department of Health (1999) *Our Healthier Nation*. Department of Health, London.
13 www.fph.org.uk (accessed 11 March 2005).
14 www.crhp.org.uk/ (accessed 11 March 2005).
15 Department of Health (2004) *Choosing Health Consultation Exercise*. Department of Health, London.
16 Roemer M (1993) Higher education for public health leadership. *Int J Health Serv*. 23: 387–400.
17 www.executive.modern.nhs.uk (accessed 28 April 2005).
18 Faculty of Public Health, NHS Leadership Centre, PHRU, BAMM (2002) Report from Workshop, May 2002, Oxford. FPH, London.
19 Griffiths S, Wright J and Thorpe A (2005) Public health in transition: views of the specialist workforce. Submitted to *Pub Health Med*.
20 Buchan J (2002) *International Recruitment of Nurses, UK Case Study*. www.rcn.org.uk/publications/pdf/irn-case-study-booklet.pdf (accessed 11 March 2005).
21 Association of Teachers of Preventive Medicine (2004) *Competency to Curriculum Toolkit – developing curricula for public health workers* (revised edn). Columbia University School of Nursing, Columbia.

22   Association of Schools of Public Health, Public Health Training Centers (2004) *Four Years of Progress in Public Health Workforce Development.* Association of Schools of Public Health, Washington, DC.

23   Hong Kong Government (2003) *Report of the SARS Expert Committee. SARS in Hong Kong: from experience to action.* www.sars-expertcom.gov.hk (accessed 11 March 2005).

24   Institute of Medicine (2002) *Who Will Keep the Public Healthy: educating public health professionals for the 21st century.* Institute of Medicine, Washington, DC. http://ilisap.rcm.upr.edu/pdfs/keep.pdf (accessed 11 March 2005).

Index

Page numbers in *italics* refer to figures or tables.

academic public health 24–6
  definitions 24
  funding and investment 25
    deficits 24
  job losses and redundancies 24
  multidisciplinary research groups 25
  and national strategic policies 25
  universities–NHS joint programmes 25
accreditation and registration 31–2, 34
'Acheson review' *see Public Health in England* (DoH 1998)
acute hospital trusts 65–6, 73–4
  public health functions and roles *23, 64,* 65–6, 74–6
    methods 76–7
    and new agenda 77–8, *77*
    specialist capacity issues 79
ADPH *see* Association of Directors of Public Health
advertising, child-targeted food adverts 10
Agenda for Change (DoH 2004) 35–6, 108
alcohol 95
Alma Ata Declaration (WHO 1978) 15, 42
appraisal frameworks 34
Association of Directors of Public Health (ADPH), on organisation models *17*
audit
  acute trusts 75
  see also health equity audit (HEA)

Balanced Score card 9, 53, 95
BAMM *see* British Association of Medical Managers
Barnard, K *et al.* 42
'Black Report' *see Report of the Working Group on Inequalities in Health* (DoH 1980)
British Association of Medical Managers (BAMM) 75–6

Canada, Public Health Agency 16
cancer registries 91
Cancer Registry staff, employing agency *22*
capacity issues *see* workforce capacity

Capacity Seminars (FPH/DoH/PHRU 2004) 98
Career Framework (Changing Workforce) 108
career structures 105–6
Centre for Applied Microbiology and Research 60
cervical screening programmes 8
Chadwick, Edwin 3
The Challenges and Opportunities for Academic Public Health (Wellcome Trust 2004) 24–5
  recommendations 25
Changing Workforce programmes 108
chief executives (CEOs) 79
Chief Medical Officer
  function and roles *22,* 74
  agenda setting 77
cholera epidemic (1832) 3–4
Choosing Health: making healthy choices easier (DoH 2004) 10, 26–7
  survey feedback on
    academic public health 25
    DPHs 'role expectations' 18
    HPA issues 66–8
    joint appointments 51
    joint targets 52–3
    role of hospitals 78–80
  and joint working/local partnership 50, 87
  key programme commitments *95*
  workforce capacity issues 26
  workforce planning 36
clinical governance 75, 77
  and public health governance 79
co-terminosity 51
Cochrane, Archie 18
Collins, Jane 76
Communicable Disease Surveillance Centre (Colindale) *23,* 60, 63
competency and career progression
  frameworks 35–6
  revalidation 32
  see also training multidisciplinary specialists

consultants in communicable disease
control (CCDCs) 18, *63*, 64
contracting arrangements 93
Council of Heads of Medical Schools 24
Council for Healthcare Regulatory
Excellence (CHRE) 109
and 'notion of equivalence' 34, 108–9

dental public health specialists 34
see also multidisciplinary specialists
Department of Health (DoH), functions
and roles of public health specialists
22
Deputy Chief Medical Officer, function
and roles *22*
directors of public health (DPHs) 47
annual report 86–7
employing agencies *22*
role 4, 10, 47
ADPH perceptions *17*
members survey 18
Donaldson, Sir Liam 77
DPHs *see* directors of public health
Duncan, William 3–4

eco-friendly initiatives, and acute sector
77
emergency planning 68
incident detection and reporting 64–5,
64
emergency response divisions *23*, 64–5
environmental health specialists *63*
epidemiology
HPA staffing *63*
public sector employers *23*
role in acute trusts 74–5
equivalence *see* 'notion of equivalence'
EU legislation 111

Faculty of Public Health (FPH) 31
on examination eligibility criteria 31
Good Public Health Practice (2001) 34
on joint working practices 43
on primary healthcare roles 43
Workforce Survey (2003) 21, 24
Fahey, D 98
flexible training 106–7
Food and Environment Water Laboratory
(FEW) *63*
FPH *see* Faculty of Public Health
funding arrangements
for academic public health 24
joint appointments 51

merged funds 90
New Opportunities Fund 9
specialist workforce career development
33, 35–6
The Future of General Practice (RCGP 2004)
43

General Medical Council (GMC),
Maintaining Good Medical Practice 34
general practice and public health 43, 49
new GP contract 47, 49, 92–3
Getting Ahead of the Curve (DoH 2002) 60
GMS contract 43, 49, 92–3
Good Public Health Practice (FPH 2001) 34
government policy *see* health policy
Great Ormond Street 76
'green hospitals' 77

health, risk factors *45*
health equity audit (HEA) 87–8
health impact assessment (HIA) 87–8
key steps 88
health improvement agenda 49
Health Information and Intelligence
Taskforce *90–1*
Health of the Nation (DoH 1992) 7
health needs surveillance *see* population
surveillance
health policy
individual choice vs. state intervention
16
key determinants of health *17*
health promotion specialists 18
health protection 59–68
incident detection and reporting 64–5,
64
see also Health Protection Agency (HPA)
Health Protection Agency (HPA) 60–8
background 59–61
consolidation of agencies 60–1
functions and roles *23*, 61, 91
key issues 64–8
key workforce sectors *63*
local and regional services (LARS) 61,
62–3
skill gaps 66–8
targets and priorities 61–2
improving emergency response 64–5,
64
vision statement 61
Healthcare Commission star ratings 87, 97
Healthy Living Centres 9
Healthy Schools Programme 8

historical background 3–7
HIV/AIDS surveillance 92
hospital trusts *see* acute hospital trusts;
        primary care trusts (PCTs)
housing conditions, background history 4
Hunt, Lord 4–5, 47

immunisation, background history 5–6
incident detection and reporting *64*
infection control *see* health protection
infection control nurses *63*
information needs, health protection 67,
        92
information sharing, and joint working
        practices 45
information technology, and surveillance
        92
Institute of Medicine 112
international working 111–12

Jackson, David 76
Jessop, E 99
Johnson, Melanie 78
joint working 44–5, *46*, 49–50
    appointments 50–2
    background 44–5
    and co-terminosity 51
    identifying vulnerable groups 45, *46*
    information sharing 45
    local strategic partnerships (LSPs) 45,
        52, 88–90
    policy directives 49–50
    target setting 52–3
    see also multidisciplinary specialists
junk food, child-targeted advertising bans
        10

Knowledge and Skills Framework (DoH
        2004) 36, 108

LARS *see* local and regional services
LDPs *see* local delivery plans
leadership 109–10
legionnaires' disease outbreak (Hereford)
        64
life-long learning 106–8
Ljubljana Charter on Reforming Health Care
        (WHO 1996) 42
local authorities and public health practice
    background 44–6
    functions and roles *23*
    joint appointments 50–2
    and co-terminosity 51

developing relationships 49–50
    funding 51
    see also local strategic partnerships (LSPs)
local delivery plans (LDPs) 87, 96–7
    and local targets 97
    performance measurement 95
Local Government Act (1929) 6
local and regional services (LARS) 61,
        62–3
    feedback on role definitions 66
    see also Health Protection Agency (HPA)
local strategic partnerships (LSPs) 45, 52,
        88–90
local target setting 52–3
London Health Observatory 87
lottery funding 8
LSPs *see* local strategic partnerships

Maintaining Good Medical Practice (GMC) 34
major incident planning *see* emergency
        planning
Maternity and Child Welfare Acts (1918) 6
medical careers *see* career structures
medical health officers (MOsH),
        background history 5–6
medical technical officers *63*
medical training
    flexibility 106–7
    Modernising Medical Careers (DoH 2004)
        35–6
    and postgraduate career structures
        105–6
    skills escalator 107–8
    see also training multidisciplinary
        specialists
Midwives Act (1902) 5
Minister for Public Health, on role of
        hospitals 78
Mitchell, G 43, *44*
Modernising Medical Careers (DoH 2004)
        35–6, 67
MRSA (methicillin-resistant *Staphylococcus
        aureus*) 61
multidisciplinary specialists 21
    training 5, 31–6, 106–8
        barriers 36
        frameworks and models *32*, 33–4
        'notion of equivalence' 34, 35, 108–9

'nanny statism' 16
National Focus for Chemical Incidents 60
National Health Service Act (1948) 6

National Institute for Health and Clinical
    Excellence (NIHCE) *22*
National Poisons Information Service 61
National Programme for Information
    Technology 92
National Radiation Protection Board *23*,
    61
National Service Frameworks (NSFs) 93–5
    need for joint working 47
    and target setting 52–3
National Standards, Local Action (DoH 2004)
    95
Neighbourhood Renewal initiatives 8
networks, supporting specialists 97–9
New Opportunities Fund 9
The NHS Improvement Plan (DoH 2004) 9,
    88–9, 93, *94*
NHS Leadership Centre 110
NHS University (NHSU) 107–8
'notion of equivalence' 34, 35, 108–9
Nuffield Institute for Health 74
nursing and midwifery public health
    specialists 34
    see also multidisciplinary specialists

obesity 95
Office for Public Management (OPM), on
    joint appointments 50, *50*
Ottawa Charter for Health Promotion (WHO
    1986) 15
Our Healthier Nation (DoH 1999) 108–9

partnership working *see* joint working
performance management 95–6
    and health equity audit (HEA) 87–8
performance measurement, health impact
    assessment 87–8
personal medical services (PMS) 93
pharmacists
    new contract 93
    as public health specialists 34
    see also multidisciplinary specialists
pharmaco-epidemiology 77
PMETB *see* Postgraduate Medical and
    Education Training Board
PMS *see* personal medical services
Pooling Resources Across Sectors (Health
    Development Agency 2004) *89*
population surveillance
    and PCT responsibilities *48*
    see also surveillance systems
Postgraduate Medical and Education
    Training Board (PMETB) 105–6

primary care and public health practice *see*
    general practice and public health;
    joint working; primary care trusts
    (PCTs)
primary care trusts (PCTs)
    and alternative providers 93
    joint appointments 50–2
    public health functions and roles 4, *23*,
        46–7, *48*
        performance management systems 9
        support networks 97–8
PSAs *see* Public Service Agreements
public health
    key domains 18
    definitions 15–16
    essential services and core functions *86*
    evaluation and performance
        management 95
    international working 111–12
    leadership 109–10
    organisational models 16–18, *17*
    see also public health specialists
public health consultants 75
Public Health in England (DoH 1998) 8, 44
    on definitions of public health 16
Public Health Laboratory Service 60
public health networks, supporting
    specialists 97–9
public health observatories 91–2
    employing agency *22*
Public Health Resource Unit (PHRU) 45
public health science *see* academic public
    health
public health service delivery,
    characteristics 18–19
public health specialists 19–20, 20–3
    key work domains 20
    background history 3–7, 21
        commissioning functions 6–7
        epidemiological focus 7
    current functions and roles *22–3*
    key areas of practice *33*
    distribution across public sector *21*
    geographical variations 21
    and leadership 109–10
    multidisciplinary agents 21
    training development 31–6
    network support 97–9
    workforce capacity 21
        acute trusts 79
        ratio to population *19*, 21
Public Health Team (DoH), function and
    roles *22*

Public Service Agreements (PSAs) targets 52, 90, 95

Quality and Outcomes Framework (QOF) 93

R&D *see* research
Raising Health (Office of Public Management 2004) 89
regional government offices, public health functions and roles *22*
registration 34–5
    development of Voluntary Register 31–2, 34–5
    and equivalence 108–9
Report of the Working Group on Inequalities in Health (DoH 1980) 7, 8
research
    in acute trusts 75
    commissioning arrangements 26
    partnership working 26
research assessment exercise (RAE), criteria on service-related work 24, 25
revalidation 32
Royal College of General Practitioners (RCGP), on GPs' role in public health 43

SARS (severe acute respiratory syndrome) 59–60, 73, 112
Saving Lives: our healthier nation (DoH 1999) 7–8
    key elements 7–8
    on multidisciplinary specialists 31
school meals
    background history 5–6
    national fruit scheme 9
school nursing, background history 5–6
Securing Good Health for the Whole Population (HM Treasury 2004) 9, 16
    on career pathways and funding 36
    on definitions of public health 16
    FPH and local government consultation 49–50
Securing Our Future: taking a long term view (HM Treasury 2002) 9–10, 42–3, 49
sexual health 95
    surveillance systems 91–2
Shifting the Balance of Power (DoH 2001)
    on DPH posts 31
    implementation 46
    on PCT's role in public health 4, 31, 46–7

skills escalator 107–8
smoking 95
    tobacco bans 10
smoking cessation programmes 8, 95
Social Exclusion Unit 8
specialist public health workforce *see* public health specialists
Specialist Training Authority 106
standards of practice 32
    appraisal frameworks 34
    see also training multidisciplinary specialists
star ratings 87, 97
strategic health authorities, public health functions and roles *22*, 65–6
SureStart 8
    targets 52
surge capacity 60, 65
surveillance systems
    and public health intelligence 90–2
    see also health protection; population surveillance
sustainability issues 77

targeted initiatives
    background to Labour policies 7–9
    Choosing Health programme commitments *95*
    and joint working 52–3
    local initiatives 97
teenage pregnancy 8
training multidisciplinary specialists 5, 31–6
    flexible packages 106–7
    frameworks 33–4
    model of training pathways *32*
    and registration 34
    skills escalator 107–8

UK Voluntary Register 31–2, 34, 108
United States 111–12
    Institute of Medicine on public health 15

Voluntary Register 31–2, 34–5, 108

'Wanless' (first) report *see Securing Our Future: taking a long term view*
'Wanless' (Second) report *see Securing Good Health for the Whole Population – final report*
Wellcome Trust, *The Challenges and Opportunities for Academic Public Health* (2004) 24–5

workforce capacity 21
   acute trusts 79
   and *Capacity Seminars* (FPH/DoH/PHRU
      2004) 98
   ratio to population *19*, 21

World Health Organization (WHO)
   Alma Ata Declaration (1978) 15, 42
   *Ljubljana Charter on Reforming Health
      Care* (1996) 42
   Ottawa Charter for Health Promotion
      (1986) 15